Parental Alienation and Family Reunification

This book on parental alienation and family reunification provides family court professionals with critical background in child development, dynamics present in violent families, and how to evaluate the testimony of experts to ensure it values children's views, best interests of the children, and follows evidence-based practice.

As laid out in the Child Welfare Information Gateway report, 2020, family court judges should make decisions per the best interests of the child standard. High conflict custody cases make this complicated, especially when reunification services are requested. In the middle of contentious proceedings, judges oftentimes receive conflicting information from parents. Judges and family law professionals can be lead astray, relying on unproven constructs and instruments not meeting the criteria of reliability and validity. Mandating victimized children into reunification programs that are neither evidence-based nor trauma-informed can cause further harm to the children.

This book will be of interest to those working in the family courts, particularly expert witnesses, clinical psychologists, therapists, children's services workers including social workers, child protection court workers, mental health professionals involved in child custody decisions, and researchers with an interest in parental alienation. The chapters in this book were originally published as a special issue of *Journal of Family Trauma, Child Custody & Child Development.*

Pearl S. Berman is Full Professor and the Chair of the Psychology Department at Indiana University of Pennsylvania, USA. She is also a licensed, clinical psychologist. Her longstanding interest in violence prevention has led her to integrate information and skill building relevant to interpersonal violence into all of her teaching at both the undergraduate and doctoral-level. She is the incoming Pennsylvania administrator for ChildFirst PA a forensic training program for first responders in cases of interpersonal violence. Berman has published doctoral-level textbooks for individuals in training to be psychologists, counselors, social workers, and therapists and has provided her research and clinical workshops nationally and internationally.

Ethan M. Weisinger is a California Certified Family Law Specialist in the San Francisco Bay Area and has practiced in family law for fourteen years. From 2010 to 2016, Ethan was a partner at Walnut Creek Family Law Center, Inc. In 2018, he founded Bay Area Family Law Center, Inc. a firm dedicated solely to the practice of family law. Ethan has lectured in the field of family law to both county and international bar associations. He served as an elected member of the Contra Costa County Bar Association, Family Law Section Board for five years. He has published articles in family law along with his monthly blog posts on family law issues. Presently, he represents clients in all conventional family law matters, as well as dissolution of Registered Domestic Partnerships and Same-Sex Marriages. Ethan also mediates and serves as a private judge in family law matters.

Parental Alienation and Family Reunification

Controversial Issues, Current Research, Approaches and Programs

Edited by
Pearl S. Berman and Ethan M. Weisinger

Routledge
Taylor & Francis Group
LONDON AND NEW YORK

First published 2024
by Routledge
4 Park Square, Milton Park, Abingdon, Oxon OX14 4RN

and by Routledge
605 Third Avenue, New York, NY 10158

Routledge is an imprint of the Taylor & Francis Group, an informa business

British Library Cataloguing in Publication Data
A catalogue record for this book is available from the British Library

ISBN13: 978-1-032-64115-7 (hbk)
ISBN13: 978-1-032-64119-5 (pbk)
ISBN13: 978-1-032-64122-5 (ebk)

DOI: 10.4324/9781032641225

Typeset in Minion Pro
by Newgen Publishing UK

Publisher's Note
The publisher accepts responsibility for any inconsistencies that may have arisen during the conversion of this book from journal articles to book chapters, namely the inclusion of journal terminology.

Contents

Citation Information

The chapters in this book were originally published in the *Journal of Family Trauma, Child Custody & Child Development*, volume 19, issue 3–4 (2022). When citing this material, please use the original page numbering for each article, as follows:

Preface

Alienation and reunification issues in family courts: Theory, research, and programs in child custody cases
Morgan Shaw and Robert Geffner
Journal of Family Trauma, Child Custody & Child Development, volume 19, issue 3–4 (2022), pp. 203–213

Introduction

Parental alienation vs coercive control: Controversial issues and current research
Pearl Berman and Ethan Weisinger
Journal of Family Trauma, Child Custody & Child Development, volume 19, issue 3–4 (2022), pp. 214–229

Chapter 1

Coercion in families and child resistance to contact with a parent after family separation
Kelly M. Champion
Journal of Family Trauma, Child Custody & Child Development, volume 19, issue 3–4 (2022), pp. 230–243

Chapter 2

"He was the king of the house" children's perspectives on the men who abused their mothers
Simon Lapierre, Isabelle Côté and Geneviève Lessard
Journal of Family Trauma, Child Custody & Child Development, volume 19, issue 3–4 (2022), pp. 244–260

Chapter 3

Examining associations between psychological control and proactive and reactive aggression among middle school age youth
Paula J. Fite, Kathleen I. Díaz and Madelaine R. Abel
Journal of Family Trauma, Child Custody & Child Development, volume 19, issue 3–4 (2022), pp. 261–273

Chapter 4

Perpetration of intimate partner violence and guilt: the role of parenting status
Emily C. Taverna, Devin J. McGuier and Amy D. Marshall
Journal of Family Trauma, Child Custody & Child Development, volume 19, issue 3–4 (2022), pp. 274–294

Chapter 5

The Trouble with Harman and Lorandos' Parental Alienation Allegations in Family Court *Study (2020)*
Joan S. Meier, Sean Dickson, Chris S. O'Sullivan and Leora N. Rosen
Journal of Family Trauma, Child Custody & Child Development, volume 19, issue 3–4 (2022), pp. 295–317

Chapter 6

Attachment issues and reunification of parents and children
Jean Mercer
Journal of Family Trauma, Child Custody & Child Development, volume 19, issue 3–4 (2022), pp. 320–339

Chapter 7

Parental sobriety and Parent-Child reunification in dependency court: Does the 15-month Adoption and Safe Families Act (ASFA) rule support parent-child reunification?
Eileen M. Ahlin, Don Hummer and Mitra Honardoost
Journal of Family Trauma, Child Custody & Child Development, volume 19, issue 3–4 (2022), pp. 340–358

Chapter 8

Reunification, alienation, or re-traumatization? Let's start listening to the child
Suzanne Chester
Journal of Family Trauma, Child Custody & Child Development, volume 19, issue 3–4 (2022), pp. 359–382

Chapter 9

Reunification therapies for parental alienation: Tenets, empirical evidence, commonalities, and differences
Jean Mercer
Journal of Family Trauma, Child Custody & Child Development, volume 19, issue 3–4 (2022), pp. 383–401

Chapter 10

How efficacious is Building Family Bridges? What the legal and mental health fields should know about Building Family Bridges and "parental alienation"
Diana S. Avalle, Brianna J. Smith, Katherine E. O. Wiedeman and Chris B. Garnica
Journal of Family Trauma, Child Custody & Child Development, volume 19, issue 3–4 (2022), pp. 402–416

Chapter 11

The "solution" to parental alienation: A critique of the turning points and overcoming barriers reunification programs
Elena Andreopoulos and Alison Wexler
Journal of Family Trauma, Child Custody & Child Development, volume 19, issue 3–4 (2022), pp. 417–437

Notes on Contributors

Madelaine R. Abel, Clinical Child Psychology Program, University of Kansas, Lawrence, KS, USA.

Eileen M. Ahlin, School of Public Affairs, Penn State Harrisburg, Middletown, PA, USA.

Elena Andreopoulos, Maastricht University, Maastricht, the Netherlands.

Diana S. Avalle, Institute on Violence, Abuse & Trauma, San Diego, CA, USA.

Pearl S. Berman, Psychology Department, Indiana University of Pennsylvania, Indiana, PA, USA.

Kelly M. Champion, Cadeus Behavioral Health, Rockville, MD, USA.

Suzanne Chester, The Child's Advocate, Legal Aid of North Carolina, Raleigh, NC, USA.

Isabelle Côté, School of Social Work, Laurentian University, Sudbury, Ontario, Canada.

Kathleen I. Díaz, Clinical Child Psychology Program, University of Kansas, Lawrence, KS, USA.

Sean Dickson, Health Policy, West Health Policy Center, Washington, D.C., USA.

Paula J. Fite, Clinical Child Psychology Program, University of Kansas, Lawrence, KS, USA.

Chris B. Garnica, Institute on Violence, Abuse & Trauma, San Diego, CA, USA.

Robert Geffner, Institute on Violence, Abuse & Trauma, San Diego, CA, USA; Psychology, Alliant International University, San Diego, CA, USA.

Mitra Honardoost, Family Preservation Unit, York County (PA) Children, Youth, and Families, York, PA, USA.

Don Hummer, School of Public Affairs, Penn State Harrisburg, Middletown, PA, USA.

Simon Lapierre, School of Social Work, University of Ottawa, Ottawa, Ontario, Canada.

Geneviève Lessard, School of Social Work, Laval University, Quebec, Quebec City, Canada.

Amy D. Marshall, Department of Psychology, The Pennsylvania State University, University Park, PA, USA.

Devin J. McGuier, Department of Psychology, The Pennsylvania State University, University Park, PA, USA; UPMC/ Children's Hospital of Pittsburgh, Pittsburgh, PA, USA.

Joan S. Meier, George Washington University Law School, Washington, D.C., USA.

Jean Mercer, Psychology Program, Department of Social and Behavioral Sciences, Stockton University, Galloway, NJ, USA.

Chris S. O'Sullivan, Research and Evaluation Consultant.

Leora N. Rosen, Independent Professional Researcher.

Morgan Shaw, Independent Practice, San Diego, CA, USA.

Brianna J. Smith, Institute on Violence, Abuse & Trauma, San Diego, CA, USA.

Emily C. Taverna, Department of Psychology, The Pennsylvania State University, University Park, PA, USA.

Ethan M. Weisinger, Bay Area Family Law Center, Inc., Walnut Creek, CA, USA.

Alison Wexler, Alliant International University, San Diego, CA, USA.

Katherine E. O. Wiedeman, Institute on Violence, Abuse & Trauma, San Diego, CA, USA.

Preface—Alienation and reunification issues in family courts: Theory, research, and programs in child custody cases

Morgan Shaw and Robert Geffner

ABSTRACT
This preface highlights the significant need for the current two-part special issue on *Alienation and Reunification Issues in Family Courts* and outlines reasons why these issues continue to be relevant. Unfortunately, there continues to be the same gross misunderstandings by legal professionals, judges, child protection workers, mental health professionals, and child custody evaluators regarding abuse dynamics and the impact of trauma on the individual. These misunderstandings then lead to many family law court cases minimizing or ignoring such issues and inferring parental alienation or similar labels instead. The impact of this on the children and families involved is great, and significant change needs to occur in the various systems involved in family law cases. This preface describes many of the main issues seen regularly in the family court system and highlights the articles included in this two-part special issue. It is hoped that the articles help address the complex issues when children resist contact with a parent, and educate evaluators, investigators, and legal decision-makers to rely on actual evidence, known research and accepted knowledge in family and trauma psychology and child development.

Over three years ago, the senior author of this preface sat at her computer contemplating how to start the introduction to a 2019 special issue on misperceptions and misapplications in family law cases, published in this same journal (Shaw, 2019). In that special issue, we covered a wide range of relevant issues including suggestibility, parental alienation, and treatment programs for youth who were reportedly "alienated" from a parent or caregiver. The goal of that special issue was to educate the courts and other relevant professionals on how to better assess and address recurrent complex issues of abuse, alienation, and estrangement arising within the family court system. At the time, we were questioned by several professionals involved in child custody cases as to the need for such a special issue since it was supposedly clear that "parental alienation syndrome" (PAS) or disorder had been debunked as junk or pseudo-science, and there was no need for the special issue. Given our experience with actual family law cases, we disagreed and went forward with the special issue.

Unfortunately, over three years later, the need for further education continues to be just as great if not more so. There continues to be the same gross misunderstandings by legal professionals, judges, child protection workers, mental health professionals, and child custody evaluators regarding abuse dynamics and the impact of trauma on adult and child victims of abuse since too many family law court cases are still minimizing or ignoring such issues and inferring parental alienation or similar labels instead. We, sadly, continue to see investigators and evaluators misunderstand and minimize indicators consistent with the effects of abuse and its resulting trauma, and to ignore disclosures of a child about abusive behaviors, poor parenting or being exposed to domestic violence. We have written about these concerns previously, but the issues are still present (e.g., Platt et al., 2016). They assign labels that are unreliable, unvalidated, nonresearched, and poorly defined, and then assert conclusions, make recommendations, and take actions based solely on these labels and supposed disorders.

They then cite outdated research studies (e.g., Ceci & Bruck, 1995) and various articles on suggestibility and coaching that are not relevant to child abuse or to the actual case (e.g., London et al., 2005), and minimize more relevant research (e.g., Goodman et al., 2009; Lyon, 2007; Saywitz et al., 2018). Many of the articles on parental alienation are anecdotal with biased and/or small samples (Baker, 2005), not methodologically sound (Harman & Lorandos, 2021), do not represent reliable "research" (Harman et al., 2022), and are not based on theory or research in the fields of family psychology, child development, or trauma psychology (Bernet, 2008; Harman et al., 2019). In fact, much of the literature supposedly supporting the dynamics of parental alienation as practiced by their proponents (still based on Gardner's outdated and unsupported principles; Gardner, 1992) contradict what is known in the fields noted above (Milchman et al., 2020). In fact, even 30 years after Gardner made up the label of PAS without any research support or reasonable operational definitions, no known mechanisms exist explaining how such indoctrination of children who supposedly have a strong relationship with a parent then leads the child to resist or refuse contact with that parent.

We repeatedly see protective parents and maltreated children further revictimized by the child protection and family court systems, often due to recommendations by child custody evaluators or mental health professionals who are not adequately trained in child development, child abuse (especially sexual abuse), domestic violence, trauma and family psychology. Regrettably, children who disclose abuse involved in the dependency system continue to be treated differently than children who disclose abuse or poor parenting who are involved in the family law system, as the latter families frequently get labeled “high conflict” and abuse disclosures are commonly dismissed by custody evaluators, mental health professionals, attorneys, including guardian ad litems (GAL), law enforcement, child protective services, and judges. With all of the research and publications in actual peer reviewed research journals concerning child abuse, domestic violence, coercive control, and trauma during the past 20 or more years (e.g., Geffner et al., 2022), we would have thought by now that these outdated and obsolete ideas and labels would have been excluded from family law cases. However, proponents of the ideas of parental alienation noted above continue to move the goal posts with their labels, to use a sports analogy, that confuses the issues and promotes junk science.

As a culture, we live currently in a time of heightened polarization across many fields and sociocultural issues, and the abuse/poor parenting versus alienation dichotomy within the family law system is no exception. Working in this field, consulting with other professionals, attending professional trainings, and reviewing professional literature, one can so clearly see the polarized camps that more frequently cited researchers, advocates, and practitioners fall into. The reality is that the polarization then trickles down to clinicians and frontline workers who carry the biases and assumptions that bleed into their work. While most professionals in these fields would likely assure others that their primary focus is first and foremost on the safety and well-being of vulnerable children, that is not how the family court system regularly acts. Instead, what we more commonly see are people who typically fall into the “pro-mother”/“pro-father” forced dichotomy, or into a forced alienation dichotomy where the provider either sees evidence of alienation in essentially every case or conversely does not acknowledge the potential for confounding factors, such as external influence, on a child.

Reflecting on where someone might place our clinical and forensic focus on those forced (and faulty) spectrums, we recognize that this problematic polarization is not outside of us or that of the colleagues with whom we more regularly align. However, self-awareness around gender biases, inappropriate assumptions, faulty inferences, appropriate training on trauma-related issues, direct experience working with trauma and abuse survivors, and a repeated re-focusing on the safety and well-being of the children are all paramount to upholding the true nature of the best interests of the child standard. It often appears that those involved in these family law cases do not pay adequate attention to the long-term effect on the children that their recommendations and decisions may have. Too often pseudo or junk science rules the day, with labels that are not supported by actual data or behavioral information being tossed around as if they do not have consequences.

Working as treatment providers, forensic evaluators, trainers, and researchers, it is intensely disappointing and frustrating how frequently investigators, evaluators, mental health professionals, and legal decision-makers are quick to discount abuse disclosures by children as evidence of coaching, despite minimal, if any, objective support for that assertion (Faller, 2007). Once the terms "alienation" or "coaching" are used in an investigative report, even without any actual evidence to support it, any subsequent disclosure or indicator of abuse or poor parenting are typically discounted and overlooked by decision-makers. One would think that law enforcement, mental health professionals, child protective services, and family court investigators would actually rely more on the evidence and records than assumptions or inferences, but our experience in evaluating cases and reports throughout the United States, Canada, and other countries, tells another story. It then puts wrongly identified protective parents in a difficult situation where they run the risk of either ongoing accusations of negative influence on their children, or conversely, fears of being labeled non-protective. We typically see the term "coaching" more commonly in investigative reports, while the terms "alienation," "enmeshment," "gate-keeping," or "resist-refuse dynamics" are more commonly seen in the reports or testimony by mental health professionals and evaluators. There are even grossly inappropriate terms that are completely misused and misunderstood in cases we have seen, such as "Munchausen by Proxy" "Factitious Disorder in Another" and many other absurd labels frequently thrown around as diagnoses when the evaluator or investigator does not want to actually say parental alienation since that is not an actual diagnosis. The use of these terms, labels, and ill-defined concepts are typically clear red flags that further assessment of abuse related issues or poor parenting by the parent the child does not want to visit is warranted.

As an example, a typical scenario in which you see these types of faulty assumptions play out in cases would be to start with a disclosure of abusive behaviors by a child concerning a parent to a trusted caregiver, such as a mother or babysitter, that is then reported to a child protective services (CPS) agency directly, or to a physician or therapist who as mandated reporters contact CPS. Following the initial report, investigative workers interview the child, and potentially a forensic interview is conducted where the child may make vague statements about being touched or may deny that anyone touches them in a way that makes them uncomfortable. The alleged perpetrator, the father in this example, denies the allegations and subsequently the investigation is closed as unfounded. The child then continues to make disclosures to the mother and/or to others, and begins to demonstrate concerning behaviors such as emotional outbursts and sexualized behaviors, but does not make clear or consistent disclosures to investigators for a variety of possible reasons. As a result of the increased stress and trauma of believing the child is being abused by their father, the mother begins to act highly distraught, comes across as disorganized, and becomes more insistent that abuse is taking place while the child is with the father. The mother may even contact an attorney at this time and file for divorce and custody of the child. The father continues to deny the allegations and tells investigators that he believes that the mother is attempting to alienate the child against him to obtain more parental time, custody, and/or money. He further highlights the "high conflict" nature of their current custody proceedings, and subsequently the investigators (e.g., CPS or law enforcement) note the child custody case, may even put this in their notes/logs, and they also begin to discount and minimize the behaviors and statements by the child. They eventually may put in their notes or logs that there are concerns of "coaching" by the mother in this scenario. The investigators also note in their records that there are concerns about the mother's mental health functioning because obviously the allegations are false even without conducting their usual thorough investigation. Too often the usual required investigation techniques and procedures that occur with children not involved in custody cases are not followed, and the assumptions of coaching and alienation become the narrative. In the above scenario, divorce was not even contemplated or filed until after repeated disclosures of abuse were made by the child, possibly also to teachers or others, and with detailed disclosures possibly beyond the child's developmental level. This timing (i.e., the disclosures occurred before any indication of divorce or custody issues) and details of the disclosures and now resistance to see that parent, in conjunction with sexualized behaviors, are often overlooked or minimized by investigators, evaluators, and courts. Circular inferences, assumptions of false allegations, perceptions, and biases have a strong influence on discounting child abuse and domestic violence in family court cases (Sanders et al. 2015; Saunders et al., 2012), and then alienation becomes the narrative.

Those notes of the CPS and law enforcement, and the poorly defined or unsupported statements about coaching and mental health concerns of the mother, continue to follow this case during the months and then years this may continue (Silberg & Dallam, 2019). The CPS records are obtained by the family law attorneys representing the family, and the statements about coaching and alienation by CPS or law enforcement begin to permeate directly into the family court. The judge who then does not know what to do with this family, decides that they are going to order a child custody evaluation, possibly with a psychosexual evaluation of the father, to hopefully rule out concern of the father engaging in sexually abusive behaviors toward his child.

Unfortunately, the family courts and too many custody evaluators misunderstand and inappropriately believe that a psychosexual evaluation on an individual who has not ever been convicted of a sex crime or admitted such behavior, and is savvy enough to know how to engage with the evaluator, will produce a meaningful result. Even more problematic is that many of the psychosexual evaluators who agree to take family law case referrals do not appropriately note the very clear limitations of their evaluations, the results, and the conclusions. For example, they do not often inform the court that such evaluations cannot rule out sexually abusive behaviors, and they may only be able to indicate such probability of offending if a person admits or fails some of the various measures or plethysmograph (e.g., Clipson, 2003; Geffner et al., 2003; Sachsenmaier, 2005). However, a sex offender, especially an incest one, can actually pass all of these measures in the evaluation. As a consequence, the results of the psychosexual evaluation may state that the father in the above scenario does not demonstrate characteristics or risk factors consistent with an individual who sexually abuses their children, as though there is a profile to actually compare this to. The investigator, or a child custody evaluator who receives this information, may then recommend that time not be limited or supervised between the father and the child, ignoring the disclosures, fears, and behaviors of the child. This faulty and very skewed result is then used in court to support increased timesharing with the father and to "prove" that the mother must be coaching and alienating the child. This may occur despite actual evidence of detailed disclosures that are not likely able to be coached, evidence of domestic violence, or confirmation of poor boundary and parenting issues by the father above. The child is then placed back into an unsafe and abusive home while time with the mother, their primary caretaker, may now be eliminated, limited and/or supervised in what has been characterized as a "parentectomy" (Geffner & Sandoval, 2020; Williams, 1990).

Unfortunately, this example is a common pattern in the cases we and many others across the country (and internationally) have seen or evaluated. We now have many examples of adults who were the unfortunate child victims of this dysfunctional and problematic system who have come forward to describe their experience. Future issues in the *Journal of Family Trauma, Child Custody, and Child Development (JFT)* will include articles concerning these situations. We have these same adults now advocating for significant change to our CPS and family court systems that so frequently fail the children and families that they are meant to serve (e.g., Cable & Riley, 2022; The Center for Investigative Reporting, 2019). We continue to have researchers and other professionals, many of whom published peer reviewed articles included in the prior special issue and now in this current special two-part issue, who are attempting to continue to educate the courts and relevant professionals about these problematic patterns and use of junk science.

It should be noted that PAS, PAD, or even parental alienation have never been successfully included in any official medical or mental health diagnostic system, despite persistent and intense promotion by the alienation activists and supporters for over 15 years in the United States and now in other countries (e.g., Crary, 2012). As we noted above about moving the goal posts, this has been the ongoing strategy by these supporters as they continue to try to change or modify labels. When PAS or Parental Alienation Disorder were denied entrance into any of the diagnostic classification systems noted above, the supporters than announced that it actually was in the classification systems under "Parent-Child Relationship Problem." The problem with this approach is that Parent-Child Relational Problem (PCRP) has been in these diagnostic codes for decades (American Psychiatric Association, 1980), having nothing to do with alienation, and even PCRP was never a diagnosis; it was labeled a behavioral issue. In moving the goal posts, they just deleted the words "syndrome" or "disorder" and just started using "alienation," attempting to couch this as child abuse or family violence in these family law cases (e.g., Harman et al., 2018). However, the principles of PAS/PAD did not change and were still the foundation of their approach and recommendations of a "parentectomy." Now the goal posts have moved once again, and these same supporters are saying that the diagnosis is actually "parent alienation relational problem" (PARP; Bernet & Baker, 2022). Keep in mind the principles have not changed, rather the label is new in an attempt to confuse people. The word "alienation" is a common lay term that most people can define. They believe it to be something one parent does to turn a child against another parent. They do not understand or know the principles, applications, and ultimately the consequences that alienation supporters promote. Regardless of how much it is promoted or the words are changed, alienation is not a research-supported clinical diagnosis. Hopefully, this sleight of hand wording will not sway the actual diagnostic classification committees.

Alienation is a behavior that could occur when one parent attempts to turn a child against another parent, as noted above. We all have had such cases, and we look for such behaviors in our evaluations or investigations. Using a common term that is familiar to all professionals and lay people makes it sound like there is objective evidence of such behaviors whenever it is used. It is actually easier to believe that a child has been alienated than it is to believe a child has been abused physically or sexually by an offending parent who does not meet any of the stereotypes of an abusive person. It is time to get back to basics in thorough investigatory evaluations no matter what the allegations are of child abuse, domestic violence or alienation (Benjamin et al., 2018; Geffner, et al., 2009). We need to look at the research, theories, behaviors, and objective evidence in these complex child custody cases. **The best interest of the child standard requires us to prioritize a child's safety and well-being.**

Thus, the current two-part special issue edited by Berman and Weisinger provide articles dealing with alternative explanations for parent alienation, such as coercive control as the key aspect of domestic violence by the parent who the child(ren) does not want to visit (Champion, 2022; Fite et al., 2022; Lapierre et al., 2022; Taverna et al., 2022). It also includes an important Commentary on challenges to research on what does happen in courts when allegations of parental alienation are promoted (Meier et al., 2022). These are the main areas of focus for Part 1 of the special issue.

The articles in Part 2 begin with reunification research in cases or situations that do not fall into the child custody cases noted in this preface. Too many evaluators use the terms of attachment or bonding without necessarily understanding what attachment research has shown, which is also discussed in one of these articles (Chester, 2022; Mercer, 2022-b). If evaluators or mental health professionals do not truly understand the attachment research, they are more likely to make mistakes in their conclusions and recommendations. Additional articles focus on the way reunification is emphasized in the alleged parental alienation cases and how they do not follow principles of known research or theory, and instead these reunification programs can produce even more trauma for these children (Chester, 2022; Mercer, 2022-b). Finally, two articles discuss the flaws and critiques of the theories and research for three major programs - Family Bridges, Turning Points, and Overcoming Barriers—utilized by parent alienation advocates and the professionals and courts who refer to them in these cases (Avalle et al., 2022; Andreopoulos & Wexler, 2022). Their critiques demonstrate the lack of adequate research or theory behind these programs and suggest they are not validated. They also discuss the ethical issues involved in the coercive methods utilized by some of these programs. These articles highlight that it is dangerous to force traumatized children into unvalidated programs that do not even refer to themselves as treatment, even when licensed mental health professionals are involved in conducting them.

Our hope is that at some point in the near future, we will no longer have the need for all of these special issues. Our goal is to no longer need to advocate so strongly for such significant change, and for the child protection and family court systems to rely on research, theory, and behavioral data that are validated and focused on the actual best interest of the children. Until then, we will continue to use these outlets to move forward the conversation and hopefully get away from false inferences, unreliable assumptions, biases, and faulty dichotomies.

Disclosure statement

The authors report no conflicts of interest. The authors alone are responsible for the content and writing of the paper.

References

American Psychiatric Association. (1980). *Diagnostic and statistical manual of mental disorders.* 3rd ed.

Andreopoulos, E., & Wexler, A. (2022). The "solution" to parental alienation: A critique of the Turning Points and Overcoming Barriers reunification programs. *Journal of Family Trauma, Child Custody & Child Development*, *19*(3/4), 417–437. https://doi.org/10.1080/26904586.2022.2049462

Avalle, D. S., Smith, B. J., Wiedeman, K. E. O., & Garnica, C. B. (2022). How efficacious is Building Family Bridges? What the legal and mental health fields should know about Building Family Bridges and "parental alienation. *Journal of Family Trauma, Child Custody & Child Development*, *19*(3/4), 402–416. https://doi.org/10.1080/26904586.2022.2066595

Baker, A. (2005). The long-term effects of parental alienation on adult children: A qualitative research study. *American Journal of Family Therapy*, *33*, 289–302. https://doi.org/10.1080/01926180590962129

Benjamin, G. A., Beck, C., Shaw, M., & Geffner, R. (2018). *Family evaluation in custody litigation: Promoting optimal outcomes and reducing ethical risks.* 2nd ed. American Psychological Association.

Bernet, W. (2008). Parental alienation disorder and DSM–V. *American Journal of Family Therapy*, *36*(5), 349–366. https://doi.org/10.1080/01926180802405513

Bernet, W., & Baker, A. (2022). (submitted June 27, Proposal for parental alienation relational problem to be included in "Other conditions that may be a focus of clinical attention" in DSM-5-TR, available at https://www.pas-intervention.org/uploads/2/2/5/4/22545256/proposal-2022-06-30.pdf

Cable, A., & Riley, A. (2022). *Protective parents in family court cases, including former youth speak out* [Paper presentation]. Keynote Panel Presentations to 27th San Diego International Summit on Violence, Abuse and Trauma across the Lifespan, La Jolla, CA. August

Ceci, S. J., & Bruck, M. (1995). Jeopardy in the courtroom: A scientific analysis of children's testimony. *American Psychological Association*, https://doi.org/10.1037/10180-000

Champion, K. (2022). Coercion in families and child resistance to contact with a parent after family separation. *Journal of Family Trauma, Child Custody & Child Development*, *19*(3/4), 230–243. https://doi.org/10.1080/26904586.2022.2105273

Chester, S. (2022). Reunification, alienation or re-traumatization? Let's start listening to the child. *Journal of Family Trauma, Child Custody & Child Development.*, *19*(3/4), 359–382. https://doi.org/10.1080/26904586.2021.1957059

Clipson, C. R. (2003). Practical considerations in the interview and evaluation of sexual offenders. *Journal of Child Sexual Abuse*, *12*(3-4), 127–173. https://doi.org/10.1300/J070v12n03_06

Crary, D. (2012). Parental alienation not a disorder, American Psychiatric Association. http://www.huffingtonpost.com/2012/09/21/parentalalienation-is-no_n_1904310.html

Faller, K. C. (2007). Coaching children about sexual abuse: A pilot study of professionals' perceptions. *Child Abuse & Neglect*, *31*(9), 947–959. https://doi.org/10.1016/j.chiabu.2007.05.004

Fite, P. J., Díaz, K. I., & Abel, M. R. (2022). Examining associations between psychological control and proactive and reactive aggression among middle school age youth. *Journal of Family Trauma, Child Custody & Child Development*, *19*(3/4), 261–273. https://doi.org/10.1080/26904586.2021.2006108

Gardner, R. A. (1992). *True and false accusations of child sex abuse*. Creative Therapeutics.

Geffner, R., Conradi, L., Geis, K., & Aranda, B. (2009). Conducting child custody evaluations in the context of family violence allegations: Practical techniques and suggestions for ethical practice. *Journal of Child Custody*, *6*(3-4), 189–218. https://doi.org/10.1080/15379410903084608

Geffner, R., Crumpton-Franey, K., Geffner-Arnold, T., & Falconer, R. (Eds.) (2003). *Identifying and treating sex offenders: Current research, approaches, and techniques*. Haworth Press.

Geffner, R., & Sandoval, A. (2020). Parental Alienation Syndrome/Parental Alienation Disorder (PAS/PAD): A critique of a 'disorder' frequently used to discount allegations of interpersonal violence and abuse in child custody cases. *APSCA Advisor*, *32*(1), 28–37.

Geffner, R., White, J. W., Hamberger, L.K., Rosenbaum, A., Vaughan-Eden, V., & Vieth, V. (Eds) (2022). *Handbook of interpersonal violence and abuse across the lifespan*. Springer Science/Nature.

Goodman, G. S., Quas, J. A., & Ogle, C. M. (2009). Child maltreatment and memory. *Annual Review of Psychology*, (61), 325–351.

Harman, J. J., Bernet, W., & Harman, J. (2019). Parental alienation: The blossoming of a field of study. *Current Directions in Psychological Science*, *28*(2), 212–217. https://doi.org/10.1177/096372141982727

Harman, J., Kruk, E., & Hines, D. (2018). Parental alienating behaviors: An unacknowledged form of family violence. *Psychological Bulletin*, *144*(12), 1275–1299. https://doi.org/10.1037/bul0000175

Harman, J., & Lorandos, D. (2021). Allegations of family violence in courts: How parental alienation affects judicial decisions. *Psychology, Public Policy, & Law*, *27*(2), 184–208. https://doi.org/10.1037/law0000301

Harman, J., Saunders, L., & Afifi, T. (2022). Evaluation of the Turning Points for Families (TPFF) program for severely alienated children. *Journal of Family Therapy*, *44*(2), 279–298. https://doi.org/10.1111/1467-6427.123666

LaPierre, S., Côté, I., & Lessard, G. (2022). "He was the king of the house." Children's perspectives on the men who abused their mothers. *Journal of Family Trauma, Child Custody & Child Development*, *19*(3/4), 1–17. https://doi.org/10.1080/26904586.2022.2036284

London, K., Bruck, M., Ceci, S., & Shuman, D. (2005). Disclosure of child sexual abuse: What does the research tell us about how children tell? *Psychology, Public Policy, and the Law*, *11*(1), 194–226. https://doi.org/10.1037/1076-8971.11.1.194

Lyon, T. D. (2007). False denials: Overcoming methodological biases in abuse disclosure research. In M. E. Pipe, M. Lamb, Y. Orbach, & A. Cederborg (Eds.), *Child sexual abuse: Disclosure, delay, and denial* (pp. 41–62). Lawrence Eribaum Associates Publishers.

Meier, J. S., Dickson, S., O'Sullivan, C., & Rosen, L. N. (2022). The trouble with Harman and Lorandos' parental alienation allegations in family court study (2020). *Journal of Family Trauma, Child Custody & Child Development, 19*(3/4), 295–317. https://doi.org/10.1080/26904586.2022.2036286

Mercer, J. (2022, a). Attachment issues and reunification of parents and children. *Journal of Family Trauma, Child Custody, & Child Development, 19*(3/4), 320–339. https://doi.org/10.1080/26904586.2021.1957055

Mercer, J. (2022, b). Reunification therapies for parental alienation: Tenets, empirical evidence, commonalities, and differences. *Journal of Family Trauma, Child Custody & Child Development, 19*(3/4), 383–401. https://doi.org/10.1080/26904586.2022.2080147

Milchman, M. S., Geffner, R., & Meier, J. S. (2020). Ideology and rhetoric replace science and reason in some parental alienation literature and advocacy: A critique. *Family Court Review, 58*(2), 340–361. https://doi.org/10.1111/fcre.12476

Platt, S., Ajami, J., Kluemper, N., Geffner, R., Shaw, M., & Assalley, A. (2016). Child protection in child custody cases: Issues and concerns. In S. Deb (Ed.), *Child safety, welfare and well-being: Issues and challenges* (pp. 313–333). Springer.

Sachsenmaier, S. J. (2005). Complex child custody evaluations: Evaluating the alleged incestuous parent. *Journal of Child Custody, 2*(3), 57–97. https://doi.org/10.1300/J190v02n03_04

Sanders, L., Geffner, R., Bucky, S., Ribner, N., & Patino, A. J. (2015). Perceptions and attitudes about intimate partner violence in child custody cases: A qualitative study of child custody evaluators' beliefs and opinions. *Journal of Child Custody, 12*(3-4), 205–230. https://doi.org/10.1080/15379418.2015.1120476

Saunders, D. G., Faller, K. C., & Tolman, R. M. (2012). *Child custody evaluators' beliefs about domestic abuse allegations: Their relationship to evaluator demographics, background, domestic violence knowledge and custody-visitation recommendations.* U.S. Department of Justice.

Saywitz, K. J., Lyon, T. D., & Goodman, G. S. (2018). When interviewing children: A review and update. In J. Conte & B. Klika (Eds.), *APSAC handbook on child maltreatment* (4th ed., pp. 310–329). Sage.

Shaw, M. (2019). Misperceptions and misapplications of research in family law cases: Myths of "Parental Alienation Syndrome" and implanted false memories. *Journal of Child Custody, 16*(1), 1–6. https://doi.org/10.1080/15379418.2019.1609384

Silberg, J., & Dallam, S. (2019). Abusers gaining custody in family courts: A case series of over turned decisions. *Journal of Child Custody, 16*(2), 140–169. https://doi.org/10.1080/15379418.2019.1613204

Taverna, E. C., McGuier, D. J., & Marshall, A. (2022). Perpetration of intimate partner violence and guilt: the role of parenting status. *Journal of Family Trauma, Child Custody, & Child Development, 19*(3/4), 274–294. https://doi.org/10.1080/26904586.2021.1994508

The Center for Investigative Reporting (2019, March 9). Bitter custody. *Reveal* [Podcast]. https://revealnews.org/podcast/bitter-custody/

Williams, F. S. (1990). *Preventing parentectomy following divorce* [Paper presentation]. Keynote Address, Fifth Annual Conference, National Council for Children's Rights, Washington, DC. October.

Introduction—Parental alienation vs coercive control: Controversial issues and current research

Pearl S. Berman and Ethan M. Weisinger

ABSTRACT
Family court judges should make decisions per the *best interests of the child standard* (Child Welfare Information Gateway, 2020). High conflict custody cases make this complicated, especially when reunification services are requested. In the middle of contentious proceedings, judges oftentimes receive conflicting information from parents. Judges and family law professionals can be lead astray, relying on unproven constructs and instruments not meeting the criteria of reliability and validity. Some victimized children have been mandated into reunification programs that are neither evidence-based nor trauma informed, causing them further harm (Chester, 2022). This two-volume special issue on Parental Alienation and Family Reunification provides courts with critical background in child development, dynamics present in violent families, and how to evaluate the testimony of experts to ensure it values children's views and follows evidence-based practice.

Introduction

Family court judges need to make decisions following the *best interests of the child standard* (Child Welfare Information Gateway, 2020). Providing for the best interest of the child in high conflict custody cases is complicated, especially when reunification services are needed. In the middle of contentious proceedings, judges oftentimes receive conflicting information from parents seeking to maintain or enhance their custodial rights. In this scenario, judges and family law professionals can easily be lead astray, relying on unproven constructs and instruments, which do not meet the criteria of reliability and validity. The American Psychological Association (APA) has put forth standards for professionals testifying in court about complex family cases that require evidence-based practices to be followed. For example, in 2013, The APA provided guidelines for psychologists completing

Psychological Evaluations in Child Protection Matters (American Psychological Association, 2013a), as well as Specialty Guidelines for Forensic Psychology (American Psychological Association, 2013b), which require professionals to only provide courts with information, evaluation methods, and treatment strategies that have undergone repeated, un-biased peer review and testing that ensures the testimony meets the best evidence-evaluable in the field.

In part, the reason for the need for evidence based, reliable therapeutic practice standards stems from concepts originating in the work of Richard Gardner. In 1992, Gardner asserted his infamous theory of Parental Alienation, hypothesizing that when there is no evidence of abuse and a child's attachment to a parent is diminished, the result might be caused by one parent poisoning the child's mind against that other parent. (Gardner 1992). Gardner's initial concept has been broadened to suggest the existence of Parental Alienation Syndrome (PAS), Parental Alienation Disorders (PAD) and/or parental alienating behaviors (PA) on the part of one parent against the other. Since 1992, several studies have been conducted to examine the validity of PAS, PAD, and PA. Unfortunately, these studies are all based on small samples, wherein the rules of experimental design, critical for valid interpretation of results, have not been followed (Saini et al., 2016).

Bowles et al. (2008) assert that PA, PAS, and PAD should not be asserted as valid concepts in court because they do not meet the criteria detailed in Daubert and Frye. The Daubert and Frye criteria require the application of a multi-factor test to any evaluation procedure used as the basis of court testimony (Cappellino, 2021). To date, the concept of PAS has not been subjected to this multifactor test and therefore the concept should not be admissible in court. The American Professional Society on the Abuse of Children (APSAC), a nonprofit, national organization focused on meeting the needs of professionals engaged in all aspects of services for maltreated children and their families, states that the concepts of PAS, PAD, PA, and Parental Alienation Behavior (PAB) give a parent's desire to have contact with a child supremacy over the child's safety (APSAC, 2012). These parental alienation concepts involve ignoring the words of the child, as the child's word is considered invalid. However, a great deal of research demonstrates that courts should listen to the words of children. Children can, and often do, provide accurate and reliable information about whether or not they have been maltreated when they are interviewed by a professional trained in child forensic evaluations (Newlin et al., 2015).

The American Professional Society on the Abuse of Children (APSAC),) (2016) has published papers on *Allegations of Interpersonal Violence in Divorce/Relationship Dissolution*, as well as *Guidelines for Forensic Evaluations*. Further, APSAC has also published *Practice Guidelines: The Investigation and Determination of Suspected Psychological Maltreatment of*

Children and Adolescents (The American Professional Society on the Abuse of Children (APSAC), 2019), that provides an in-depth evaluation of sexual abuse cases wherein a child has disclosed sexual abuse in the context of a divorce or custody dispute. In addition, the National Institute of Child Health and Human Development (Hershkowitz et al., 2007) and the Zero Abuse Project (Farrell & Vieth, 2020) have structured interview protocols that provide step-by-step guidelines for interviewing children about potential abuse and violence to gain accurate responses.

One major bias that many family law professionals maintain is the belief that a child's and/or a parent's delay in disclosing abuse indicates that the abuse allegations are not based on fact. While some children delay disclosure of abuse until a custody dispute begins, Faller (2020) and The American Professional Society on the Abuse of Children (APSAC) (2019) discuss the issues that might cause these delays in disclosure. In addition, there are documented cases wherein perpetrators of maltreatment have threatened a child to prevent disclosure, have bribed a child not to disclose, or cases where the child fears causing distress to the supportive parent. Non-disclosure might be the most common response to child maltreatment based on studies in Israel and Canada (Hershkowitz et al., 2005; Pipe et al., 2007).

Volume 1

Some biological parents do not have adequate parenting skills and some use techniques, like coercive control, that are harmful to a developing child. Kelly Champion, in this volume, in her article "Coercion in Families and Child Resistance to Contact with a Parent After Family Separation" provides the background needed to understand the research literature currently available for understanding and changing children's resistance or refusal to follow the requests of their parents (Champion, 2022).

She reviews the behavior of parents that has led to poor parent-child relationships. Sometimes these poor relations are caused by parents who use coercive control, a form of emotional abuse, and other forms of child abuse and/or intimate partner violence that are harmful to child development. The article concludes with underscoring the critical need for family courts to have comprehensive evaluations completed by professionals who understand coercive control and abusive family practices. Such a background in the evaluator is needed in order to more fully understand family dynamics and provide judges with the information they need to make rulings that are in the *best interests of the child.*

Critical to Gardner's original conception of "parental alienation" was the idea that a comprehensive assessment had been completed to rule out the possibility that child rejection of a parent was due to family violence, coercion, or neglect. The need for a comprehensive assessment is underscored by the work of Tomlinson et al. (2019). Studies on disclosure (Faller, 2020; Hershkowitz et al., 2007; Newlin et al., 2015; Pipe et al., 2007) indicate that common patterns of disclosure can include delayed disclosure, recanted disclosure, and perhaps 60-80% do not disclose until adulthood (Alaggia, 2010). These disclosure patterns indicate that children not spontaneously disclosing abuse prior to a custody dispute do not mean that their lack of interest in seeing a parent was due to parental alienation.

Meier and Dickson (2017) concluded that family law professionals should strive to be aware of the bias inherent in the legal profession when one parent raises issues of abuse, while the other parent raises issues of alienation. Claims of alienation should not diminish nor refute the alleged-alienator's claim that domestic violence has occurred in the family home. Judges especially should be aware that not all domestic violence is reported. Furthermore, when cases go to court and agree to voluntary Alternate Dispute Resolution (ADR) mediation to try and settle issues of child custody, over 50% of these families have reported intimate partner violence; a concern in mediation is that one partner enters the mediation due to coercion of the other partner. A divorce or separation itself does not prevent future acts of violence between the adults. McTavish et al. (2016) found that children exposed to intimate partner violence may experience serious internalizing problems such as anxiety, depression, sleep disturbances, as well as externalizing disturbances such as aggression, juvenile delinquency, and Post Traumatic Stress Disorder.

Why coercive control and direct violence can lead to an insecure attachment or a breach in attachment with one parent, and make the children's welfare completely dependent on another, can be understood through the article in this volume by LaPierre, Côté & Lessard, "He was the King of the House: Children's perspectives on men who abused their mothers." This article provides important background on the impact of living in male-caused intimate partner violence, and how it influences the behavior of the children and the supportive parent. The article further explores how children's relationships with their parents are affected by domestic violence. The Canadian Social Sciences and Humanities Research Council funded Lapierre's work which gives voice to the perspectives of children (See Lapierre, 2022). Children expressed living with violence and coercive control and this evoked many negative feelings in them. Most of the children reported being relieved that they no longer had to see their fathers or had only limited contact with him. There were some children who indicated that their relationship with their fathers improved once the divorce had taken place.

Fite, Díaz, and Abel (2022) in their article, "Examining Associations between Psychological Control and Proactive and Reactive Aggression among Middle School Age Youth" discuss how parents using psychological control such as guilt or love withdrawal to manipulate children's behavior can lead to increased aggression. There was an increase in both proactive and reactive aggression, however, the impact was greatest in boys and for reactive aggression. In this form of aggression, the behavior is an impulsive reaction to being teased or threatened. While the authors had expected levels of anxiety to mediate aggression, this was not found to be the case.

Next, in "Perpetration of Intimate Partner Violence and Guilt: the Role of Parenting Status", Taverna, McGuier & Marshall explore intimate partner violence (IPV) and the role of guilt in family systems. In contrast to their hypothesis, they found that moral emotions such as guilt following perpetration of IPV were more common in non-parents than in parents. This preliminary study supports a need for IPV prevention and intervention programs to address moral emotions. According to the authors, reduced feelings of guilt following IPV perpetration among parents "may limit their motivation to change their behavior….thereby increasing risk for future perpetration." More research is needed in this area to reduce future perpetration as children's exposure to IPV can lead to a variety of negative outcomes (Artz et al., 2014 in Taverna et al., 2022).

Meier, Dickson, O'Sullivan & Rosen have contributed a commentary titled, "The Trouble with Harman and Lorandos' Parental Alienation Allegations in Family Court Study (2020)". This work analyzes an article by Harman and Lorandos, illustrating that the arguments by these authors are grounded in design and methodological errors. Lastly, volume 1 of this special edition ends with a review by Kohutis of the book, "Challenging parental alienation: New directions for professionals and parents" edited by Jean Mercer and Margaret Drew (2022), that may be helpful for professionals in the field to consider reading (See Kohutis, 2022). Written by an international group of known scholars in the fields of psychology and law, the publication discusses various reasons a child may reject – or resist – the other parent, and addresses controversies "that other sources avoid."

Volume 2

Developmental psychology is a broad field with a vast literature on children, youth, and families. Within this literature, attachment has been broadly studied and has been found to change with developmental stages of children and adolescents. Family court judges and court personnel need to understand how healthy parent-child attachments are formed, how they develop over time, and whether it is likely that a child or adolescent would reject a parent with whom they had a secure attachment without the rejection being based on child abuse, neglect or intimate partner violence. How susceptible/vulnerable are children to being manipulated by a parent to turn away from their attachment with the other parent? These are all considerations that are critical for family judges and judicial personnel to understand. Jean Mercer in her article in this issue, "Attachment issues and Reunification of Parents and Children," addresses these important issues. When Judges wish to understand a relationship between a parent and a child, it is critical that the child's point of view is given serious consideration (Mercer, 2022). Meier and Dickson (2017) found that when mothers brought allegations of child sexual abuse to the attention of the court, and the father countered with allegations of parental alienation, in only 6% of cases were the child's claims credited. However, research has consistently shown that children typically tell the truth and that false allegations only represent a small percentage of the population (Faller, 1984; Lyon & Dorado, 2008; O'Donohue et al., 2018; Ruck, 1996; Rush, 2014).

Mercer's article draws on the broad research literature on the developmental needs of children and adolescents, and the immediate and long-term negative impact of exposure to child abuse, neglect, sexual abuse, and intimate partner violence. Her article can offer guidance to parenting plans and reunification efforts that involve infants and young children within specific age groups from infancy, toddlerhood, preschoolers and kindergarteners, school-age children and adolescents. She then proceeds to discuss how attachment theory should be used to ensure the best interests of the child are being met by promoting healthy attachments with caregivers instead of improperly using attachment theory as the basis for an order that a child must have contact with a parent, even in the face of abuse allegations. She draws attention to how so called "reunification therapies" misuse the concept of attachment. She concludes with information on how family preservation and/or reunification could be addressed appropriately within high conflict divorces; these efforts are often dependent on the adults within the family circle being willing to gain the therapeutic resources or parenting skills that they need to form healthy relationships with their children. Understanding the basic needs of children to form positive and secure attachments is important for all family court judges. Further, judges need to understand the difference between a child's healthy attachments and a connection that only exists due to biology.

Child Protective Services must place children in foster care when their parents are temporarily not able to provide them with adequate care due to substance abuse. When is it safe for the children to be returned home?

If it is taking too long for parents to become free of substances, should their parental rights be terminated? Ahlin, Hummer & Honardoost (2022) examine these issues in their article, "Parental Sobriety and Parent-Child Reunification in Dependency Court: Does the Adoption and Safe Families Act Support Parent-Child Reunification?". The authors examine whether the Adoption and Safe Families Act (ASFA) of 1997 has resulted in children gaining secure home environments faster than they had in the past. Results showed that children were less likely to be reunited with their parents when abuse and/or neglect was also at issue in addition to substance abuse. The authors also found that older children were more likely to be reunited with parents than younger ones.

Judges would benefit from knowing about evidence-based and trauma-informed treatments that could help the families coming before them. The next section in this issue will discuss the issue of reunification and explore programs that have been promoted as showing effectiveness in helping in healthy reunification. First in this issue section, Suzanne Chester lays a foundation about issues with reunification in her article, "Reunification, alienation or re-traumatization? Let's start listening to the child." She illustrates how forcing contact with a parent who has legitimate reasons for not wanting this contact can lead to further harm to a child. In the case used as an example, the child was sexually abused by her father who was seeking forced contact with her. Chester uses this case to make concrete the pain and suffering caused by a court ordering reunification therapy to combat "parental alienation." The litigation involving a 12-year-old girl is discussed. Reports made to Child Protective Services led to a substantiated case of sexual abuse by the father, but this is then reversed by the courts allowing abuse to continue. Later investigations documented the child being harmed by pets in his home and his neglect of the child's safety, which led to visitation being temporarily discontinued. Despite later new allegations of sexual abuse that were founded, the girl was still forced to participate in reunification therapy. The APA does not include reunification therapy as evidenced-based or trauma-informed (Kleinman, 2017). In the final court case that forms the conclusions of this article, the family court judge was presented with the testimony of many experts, thus having a great deal of background information to digest. The judge was facing a very difficult situation when trying to decide who and what to believe. The article provides guidelines derived from what happened in this case that could be invaluable to family court judges. These guidelines include how to make decisions about which experts are considered to be qualified to testify for the particular issues facing the court as well as which types of evidence carry the weight of reliability and validity and are backed up by the weight of most professionals in the field.

The next article by Mercer, "Reunification therapies for Parental Alienation: Tenets, empirical evidence, commonalities, and differences," explores six different intensive reunification programs, and describes some of the shared tenets and assumptions amongst them. Mercer carefully and thoroughly critiques the tenets, treatment methods, and outcomes of each program. She concludes that many program tenets are questionable and that outcome studies are too weakly designed and implemented to provide evidence of the programs' effectiveness. Further information is provided that can be used by courts in understanding more of how these programs are being used.

Divorce and child custody cases often have litigants who are struggling financially, which limits their ability to hire an attorney to represent their wishes in court, as well as their ability to pay for treatment resources that the court might mandate. A highly expensive and well- regarded program within the proponents of parent alienation treatment programs is the Building Family Bridges program. The article by Avalle, Smith, Wiedeman & Garnica titled, "How efficacious is Building Family Bridges? What the legal and mental health fields should know about Building Bridges and "parental alienation," describes the parental alienation treatment camps, wherein the ultimate goal of the treatment camps is to reestablish the relationship between the child(ren) and the targeted parent. This is done typically by completely removing the child(ren) from the preferred parent and oftentimes granting full custody to the targeted parent. The children undergo treatment with the alienated parent to try to give the children perspective about the tactics of the alienating parent and to show the alienated children that their feelings against the alienated parent may not be justified after reviewing the facts of the child's shift from a healthy relationship with the alienated parent to an unhealthy relationship. The article describes the techniques and tactics of the Building Family Bridges Program. The article concludes that these programs require further unbiased peer review. Legal professionals should again be aware of the hefty price tag of these programs as well as the danger of trauma in cases where an attempted reunification occurs in the face of undisclosed domestic violence. Family Bridges is the largest program of its kind in North America, but it operates outside the mainstream of psychological treatment. Until recently, it had no website; its four-day workshops take place in hotels and resorts, and they're not cheap. The minimum fee is $20,000, but add to that room, board, transportation for family members—and, sometimes, the cost of hiring security personnel to escort resistant children—and the tab can run upwards of $30,000 (Hagerty, 2020).

The next article in Volume 2 is, "The 'Solution' to Parental Alienation: A Critique of the Turning Points and Overcoming Barriers Reunification

Programs," by Andreopoulus & Wexler. This article describes Linda Gottlieb's *Turning Points* (New York, New York; Austin, Texas) as well as Deutsch, Ward, Sullivan, and Friend's *Overcoming Barriers* (Palo Alto, California; Natick, Massachusetts; New York, New York) (Andreopoulos & Wexler, 2022). Both programs are multi-day educational programs with the child and alienated parent, which remove the child for a period from the alienating parent. The authors conclude that efficacy of the programs requires further unbiased peer review. Two drawbacks to these programs are: (1) these programs carry hefty price tags and (2) a referral to these programs in the face of undisclosed domestic violence may present a danger of traumatizing the minor child by the program's emphasis that the child should reunify with the alienated-parent. In the face of domestic violence, such a result could be detrimental to the minor child.

Conclusions from Volume 1 and 2

Richard Gardner (1985) proposed PAS as an explanation of cases where children showed no interest in having a relationship with one of their parents and there was clearly no maltreatment at issue. Since then, there has been a burgeoning interest in this explanatory possibility within some experts who testify in court using this explanation and some courts making decisions based on it being accurate despite there being no reliable and valid research base in support of a syndrome construct or symptoms of PA. In addition, there is a research base indicating there is a low rate of false allegations of children being maltreated by divorcing parents (Orchowski et al., 2020; Petherick, 2019) and the commonness of children giving delayed disclosures in cases of sexual abuse by a parent (Hershkowitz et al., 2007).

A valuable recommendation for family court judges, weighing the evidence within high conflict divorce cases when abuse or violence have been raised, would be to require a friend of the court evaluation including a comprehensive evaluation for family violence relying on interviews with all adults and children in the case and involving use of only testing protocols that have undergone considerable research, the test of time, have the support of professional organizations with expertise in children and youth, and that collect extensive background on the children's past development. An example of a reliable, valid, and well-regarded protocol is the National Institute of Child Health and Human Development (NICHD) Investigative Interview Protocol. In addition to being a highly regarded instrument for use in ongoing cases, it has also been used in basic research on issues relevant to child abuse and neglect. For example, this protocol has helped develop the research base on when children do or do not make disclosures of abuse (Newlin et al., 2015). Using this structured interview, examiners found that delayed disclosures of sexual abuse were common. More than half of their sample, 53% did not disclose until 1 week to 2 years after sexual maltreatment. For the children who showed delayed disclosure, 78% were familiar with the perpetrator. If the offenses were severe, then 92% showed delayed disclosure. One third of those who showed delayed disclosure indicated being threatened by the perpetrator and 23% were given rewards with emotional significance if they agreed to keep sexual abuse a secret; yet a third group were trying to protect their non-abusive parent from distress.

Experts who seek to testify in high-conflict divorce cases that have allegations of child abuse, neglect, or intimate partner violence need to have a background that includes a thorough grounding in child development and the impact of violence and/or coercive control on family dynamics. National surveys supported by The Department of Justice have found that in court cases without essential expertise in these areas, professionals were more likely to believe allegations of parental alienation over child maltreatment (Milchman, 2020). Unfortunately, family court judges have been shown to credit the explanations provided by PA, PAD, and PAS claims despite their lack of real validity (Meier & Dickson, 2017). This has led to decisions where the protective parent has lost custody to the parent that children alleged to have abused them; this type of decisions causes further psychological damage to children who have already been harmed.

Judges cannot be experts in every issue that is likely to come before them in family court. Therefore, it is critical that they know how to evaluate the depth of the expert's knowledge in the areas they are testifying about. For cases in which allegations of family violence have been made, the judge must be able to assess: (1) how deep the expert's grounding is in the research and treatment of abused children and violent families, (2) how thoroughly the expert is trained in how to talk to and understand what children and adolescents said during evaluations they performed and, (3) how much the expert's testimony is based on the use of validated, structured protocols respected in the field of family violence for evaluating the present or absence of child maltreatment (Conte & Simon, 2020). Judges must also understand that mistakenly applying the term "parental alienation" to families in which some form of family violence has taken place can lead to further traumatization of children and youth who have already been harmed by serious parental misconduct. It is possible that a child or adolescent could lose interest in contact with a parent for reasons that could be overcome such as a parent being absent for a long period of time or a parent getting treatment for a problem, such as an addiction, that had made them a neglectful parent in the past. However, prior to making judicial orders that consider PA something that can be overcome with treatment services, violence in all its forms must be ruled out first.

The best *interests of the child* or *children's rights* have been examined in many countries around the world (Keddell, 2017). Standards for the *best interest of the child* include two major components. One is that children have their own psychological needs which are separate from those of the parent. The second is that children have evolving capacities, and the needs of the child do not always match the needs of adults who want relationships with them (Galeş & Florea, 2021). Children have the right to have experiences that allow for their full physical, psychological, and moral development so that they can relate to adults and other children within a physically and psychological secure environment.

If there is a history of child abuse, neglect, or any other form of violence, the possibility of future risk for violence must be taken seriously. If there is a problem in the parent-child relationship, it is the parents who must take steps to change through increasing their understanding of child development and learning to set boundaries between what they want and providing minors with what they need (Galeş & Florea, 2021). The Multidimensional Assessment Protocol (MAP) is an example of an approach that could help identify which of a variety of important reasons might be behind a child indicating they did not want to live with or visit a parent (Milchman, 2020). The APSAC Practice Guidelines: The Investigation and Determination of Suspected Psychological Maltreatment of Children and Adolescents (The American Professional Society on the Abuse of Children (APSAC), 2019) helped inform MAP. This includes issues such as history of bad parenting, psychological maltreatment, child sexual abuse and/or other forms of maltreatment, and PA. Comprehensive assessments by a qualified forensic interviewer are critical to providing family court judges with the information they need *to listen fully to the child* and make decisions in *the best interests of the child.*

Parents who have used any form of violence or coercive control within family life are responsible for any damage they may have done to parent-child relationships (Tomlinson et al., 2020) and must be held accountable for this in child custody and/or visitation arrangements. The Battered Women's Justice Project (Davis et al., 2018) provides research-informed guidelines that family courts can use in making decisions in cases where there has been intimate partner violence.

Successful building of relationships come from the adults showing meaningful engagement in raising their awareness of the impact of their past behavior on their children and developing skills needed to work toward attempting to rebuild a healthy parent-child relationship. In this process, it should be based on the child's wishes, not those of the parent, if attempts at reunification occur. There are already evidence-based treatments available to help adults learn better parenting skills and/or help children who have experienced maltreatment to recover without risk of future re-traumatization. These include the Triple P-Positive Parenting Program (Nowak & Heinrichs, 2008; Prinz et al., 2009; Sanders et al. 2008), Parent Child Interaction Therapy (Chronis-Tuscano et al., 2016; Kaminski & Claussen, 2017; Karoly & Auger, 2016), and Multi-Systemic Treatment (Butler et al., 2011; Timmons-Mitchell et al., 2006; Zajac et al., 2015). There is no need for family court justices to send children and youth for specialized treatments designed specifically for issues of "alienation" prior to these specialized treatments undergoing the same rigorous, peer-evaluated processes as other forms of treatment already found effective for a diverse range of parent-child problems.

Acknowledgments

In collaboration with the National Partnership to End Interpersonal Violence Across the Lifespan (NPEIV).

Disclosure statement

The authors report no conflicts of interest. The authors alone are responsible for the content and writing of the paper.

References

Ahlin, E. M., Hummer, D., & Honardoost, M. (2022). Parental sobriety and Parent-Child reunification in dependency court: Does the 15-month Adoption and Safe Families Act (ASFA) rule support parent-child reunification? *Journal of Family Trauma, Child Custody & Child Development*, *19*(3/4), 340–358. https://doi.org/10.1080/26904586.2021.1957060

Alaggia, R. (2010). An ecological analysis of child sexual abuse disclosure: Considerations for child and adolescent mental health. *Journal of the Canadian Academy of Child and Adolescent Psychiatry*, *19*(1), 32–39.

American Psychological Association. (2013a). Guidelines for psychological evaluations in child protection matters. *American Psychologist*, *68*(1), 20–31. https://doi.org/10.1037/a0029891

American Psychological Association. (2013b). Specialty guidelines for forensic psychology. *American Psychologist*, *68*(1), 7–19. https://doi.org/10.1037/a0029889

Andreopoulos, E., & Wexler, A. (2022). The “solution” to parental alienation: A critique of the turning points and overcoming barriers reunification programs. *Journal of Family Trauma, Child Custody & Child Development*, *19*(3/4), 417–437. https://doi.org/10.1080/26904586.2022.2049462

Avalle, D. S., Smith, B. J., Wiedeman, K. E. O., & Garnica, C. B. (2022). How efficacious is Building Family Bridges? What the legal and mental health fields should know about Building Family Bridges and "parental alienation. *Journal of Family Trauma, Child Custody & Child Development*, *19*(3/4), 402–416. https://doi.org/10.1080/26904586.2022.2066595

Bowles, J. J., Christian, K. K., Drew, M. B., & Yetter, K. L. (2008). *A judicial guide to child safety in custody cases*. National Association of Juvenile and Family Court Judges. https://www.ncjfcj.org/wp-content/uploads/2012/02/judicial-guide_0_0.pdf

Butler, S., Baruch, G., Hickey, N., & Fonagy, P. (2011). A randomized controlled trial of multisystemic therapy and a statutory therapeutic intervention for young offenders. *Journal of the American Academy of Child & Adolescent Psychiatry*, *50*(12), 1220–1235.e2. https://doi.org/10.1016/j.jaac.2011.09.017

Cappellino, A. (2021). *Daubert vs. frye: Navigating the standards of admissibility for expert testimony*. Expert Institute. https://www.expertinstitute.com/resources/insights/daubert-vs-frye-navigating-the-standards-of-admissibility-for-expert-testimony/

Champion, K. (2022). Coercion in families and child resistance to contact with a parent after family separation. *Journal of Family Trauma, Child Custody & Child Development*, *19*(3/4), 230–243. https://doi.org/10.1080/26904586.2022.2105273

Chester, S. (2022). Reunification, alienation or re-traumatization? Let's start listening to the child. *Journal of Family Trauma, Child Custody & Child Development*, *19*(3/4), 359–382. https://doi.org/10.1080/26904586.2021.1957059

Child Welfare Information Gateway. (2020). Determining the best interests of the child. https://www.childwelfare.gov/pubpdfs/best_interest.pdf

Chronis-Tuscano, A., Lewis-Morrarty, E., Woods, K. E., O'Brien, K. A., Mazursky-Horowitz, H., & Thomas, S. R. (2016). Parent–child interaction therapy with emotion coaching for preschoolers with attention-deficit/hyperactivity disorder. *Cognitive and Behavioral Practice*, *23*(1), 62–78. https://doi.org/10.1016/j.cbpra.2014.11.001

Conte, J. R., & Simon, J. (2020). Sexual abuse of children. In R. Geffner, J. W. White, L. K. Hamberger, A. Rosenbaum, V. Vaughan-Eden, & V. I. Vieth (Eds.), *Handbook of interpersonal violence and abuse across the lifespan*. Springer. https://doi.org/10.1007/978-3-319-62122-7_100-1

Davis, G., Frederick, L., & Steegh, N. V. (2018). Practice guides for family court decision-making in domestic abuse-related child custody matters. Battered Women's Justice Project. Retrieved from: https://www.bwjp.org/assets/compiled-practice-guides-may-2018.pdf

Faller, K. C. (1984). Is the child victim of sexual abuse telling the truth? *Child Abuse & Neglect*, *8*(4), 473–481. https://doi.org/10.1016/0145-2134(84)90029-2

Faller, K. C. (2020). The child sexual abuse disclosure controversy: New perspectives on an abiding problem. *Child Abuse & Neglect*, *99*(1), 104285. https://doi.org/10.1016/j.chiabu.2019.104285

Farrell, R., & Vieth, V. (2020). ChildFirst forensic interview training program. Retrieved April 22, 2022, from http://apsaclibrary.org/publications/2020%20Number%202/10566.pdf

Fite, P. J., Díaz, K.I., & Abel, M. R. (2022). Examining associations between psychological control and proactive and reactive aggression among middle school age youth. *Journal of Family Trauma, Child Custody & Child Development*, *19*(3/4), 261–273. https://doi.org/10.1080/26904586.2021.2006108

Galeş, N., & Florea, D. (2021). Best interests of the child – The legal determination of the principle. *European Journal of Law and Public Administration*, *8*(2), 15–25. https://doi.org/10.18662/eljpa/8.2/156

Gardner, R. (1985). Recent trends in divorce and custody litigation. *Academy Forum*, *29*(2), 3–7.

Gardner, R. (1992). *The parental alienation syndrome* (2nd ed.). Creative Therapeutics.

Hagerty, B. B. (2020). Can children be persuaded to love a parent they hate? *The Atlantic*. https://www.theatlantic.com/magazine/archive/2020/12/when-a-child-is-a-weapon/616931/

Hershkowitz, I., Horowitz, D., & Lamb, M. E. (2005). Trends in children's disclosure of abuse in Israel: A national study. *Child Abuse & Neglect*, *29*(11), 1203–1214. https://doi.org/10.1016/j.chiabu.2005.04.008

Hershkowitz, I., Lanes, O., & Lamb, M. E. (2007). Exploring the disclosure of child sexual abuse with alleged victims and their parents. *Child Abuse & Neglect*, *31*(2), 111–123. https://doi.org/10.1016/j.chiabu.2006.09.004

Kaminski, J. W., & Claussen, A. H. (2017). Evidence base update for psychosocial treatments for disruptive behaviors in children. *Journal of Clinical Child and Adolescent Psychology: The Official Journal for the Society of Clinical Child and Adolescent Psychology, American Psychological Association, Division 53*, *46*(4), 477–499. https://doi.org/10.1080/15374416.2017.1310044

Karoly, L. A., & Auger, A. (2016). *Informing investments in preschool quality and access in Cincinnati: Evidence of impacts and economic returns from national, state, and local preschool programs*. RAND Corporation.

Keddell, E. (2017). Interpreting children's best interests: Needs, attachment, and decision-making. *Journal of Social Work*, *17*(3), 324–342. https://doi.org/10.1177/1468017316644694

Kleinman, T. (2017). Family court ordered "reunification therapy": junk science in the guise of helping parent/child relationships? *Journal of Child Custody*, *14*(4), 295–300. https://doi.org/10.1080/15379418.2017.1413699

Kohutis, E. A. (2022). Challenging parental alienation: New directions for professionals and parents. *Journal of Family Trauma, Child Custody & Child Development*. https://doi.org/10.1080/26904586.2022.2112359

Lapierre, S., Côté, I., & Lessard, G. (2022). He was the king of the house." Children's perspectives on the men who abused their mothers. *Journal of Family Trauma, Child Custody & Child Development*, *19*(3/4), 244–260. https://doi.org/10.1080/26904586.2022.2036284

Lyon, T. D., & Dorado, J. S. (2008). Truth induction in young maltreated children: The effects of oath-taking and reassurance on true and false disclosures. *Child Abuse & Neglect*, *32*(7), 738–748. https://doi.org/10.1016/j.chiabu.2007.08.008

McTavish, J. R., MacGregor, J. C. D., Wathen, C. N., & MacMillan, H. L. (2016). Children's exposure to intimate partner violence: An overview. *International Review of Psychiatry*, *28*(5), 504–518. https://doi.org/10.1080/09540261.2016.1205001

Meier, J., & Dickson, S. (2017). Mapping gender: Shedding empirical light on family courts' treatment of cases involving abuse and alienation. *Journal of Child Custody, Law and Inequality*, *35*(2), 311–334.

Meier, J. S., Dickson, S., O'Sullivan, C., & Rosen, L. N. (2022). The trouble with Harman and Lorandos' parental alienation allegations in family court study (2020). *Journal of Family Trauma, Child Custody & Child Development*, *19*(3/4), 295–317. https://doi.org/10.1080/26904586.2022.2036286

Mercer, J. (2022-a). Attachment issues and reunification of parents and children. *Journal of Family Trauma, Child Custody, & Child Development*, *19*(3/4), 320–339. https://doi.org/10.1080/26904586.2021.1957055

Mercer, J. (2022-b). Reunification therapies for parental alienation: Tenets, empirical evidence, commonalities, and differences. *Journal of Family Trauma, Child Custody & Child Development*, *19*(3/4), 383–401. https://doi.org/10.1080/26904586.2022.2080147

Milchman, M. S. (2020). Assessing causes of children's parent rejection in child custody cases: Differentiating parental alienation from child sexual abuse, psychological maltreatment, and bad parenting. *Handbook of Interpersonal Violence and Abuse across the Lifespan*, 1–21. https://doi.org/10.1007/978-3-319-62122-7_318-1

Newlin, C., Steele, L. C., Chamberlin, A., Anderson, J., Kenniston, J., Russell, A., Stewart, H., & Vaughan-Eden, V. (2015). *Child forensic interviewing: Best practices*, Juvenile Justice Bulletin [NCJ 248749], U.S. Department of Justice, Office of Justice Programs, Office of Juvenile Justice and Delinquency Prevention, 1–17. https://ojjdp.ojp.gov/sites/g/files/xyckuh176/files/pubs/248749.pdf

Nowak, C., & Heinrichs, N. (2008). A comprehensive meta-analysis of Triple P-Positive Parenting Program using hierarchical linear modeling: Effectiveness and moderating variables. *Clinical Child and Family Psychology Review*, *11*(3), 114–144. https://doi.org/10.1007/s10567-008-0033-0

O'Donohue, W., Cummings, C., & Willis, B. (2018). The frequency of false allegations of child sexual abuse: A critical review. *Journal of Child Sexual Abuse*, *27*(5), 459–475. https://doi.org/10.1080/10538712.2018.1477224

Orchowski, L., Bogen, K. W., & Berkowitz, A. (2020). False reporting of sexual victimization: Prevalence, definitions, and public perceptions. In R. Geffner, J. W. White, L. K. Hamberger, A. Rosenbaum, V. Vaughan-Eden, & V. I. Vieth (Eds.), *Handbook of interpersonal violence and abuse across the lifespan*. Springer. https://doi.org/10.1007/978-3-319-62122-7_193-1

Petherick, W. (2019). False reports in child abuse and neglect cases. In I. Bryce, Y. Robinson, & W. Petherick (Eds.), *Child abuse and neglect: Forensic issues in evidence, impact, and management* (pp. 263–287). Elsevier Academic Press. https://doi.org/10.1016/B978-0-12-815344-4.00014-3

Pipe, M.-E., Lamb, M. E., Orbach, Y., Sternberg, K. J., Stewart, H. L., & Esplin, P. W. (2007). Factors associated with nondisclosure of suspected abuse during forensic interviews. In M-E. Pipe, M.E. Lamb, Y. Orbach, & A-C. Cederborg (Eds.), *Child sexual abuse: Disclosure, delay, and denial*. Routledge, Taylor & Francis Group.

Prinz, R. J., Sanders, M. R., Shapiro, C. J., Whitaker, D. J., & Lutzker, J. R. (2009). Population-based prevention of child maltreatment: the U.S. Triple p system population trial. *Prevention Science: The Official Journal of the Society for Prevention Research*, *10*(1), 1–12. https://doi.org/10.1007/s11121-009-0123-3

Ruck, M. D. (1996). Why children think they should tell the truth in court: Developmental considerations for the assessment of competency. *Legal and Criminological Psychology*, *1*(1), 103–116. https://doi.org/10.1111/j.2044-8333.1996.tb00310.x

Rush, E. (2014). Children's true and false disclosures of transgressions: Balancing costs and benefits of a novel interviewing technique. In *Dissertation abstracts international: Section B: The sciences and engineering*. University of California.

Saini, M., Johnston, J., Fidler, B., & Bala, N. (2016). Empirical evidence of alienation: Updated review. In L. Drozd, M. Saini, & N. Olesen (Eds.), *Parenting plan evaluations: Applied research for the family court* (2nd ed.). Oxford University Press.

Sanders. (2008).

Taverna, E. C., McGuier, D. J., & Marshall, A. D. (2022). Perpetration of intimate partner violence and guilt: the role of parenting status. *Journal of Family Trauma, Child Custody, & Child Development*, *19*(3/4), 274–294. https://doi.org/10.1080/26904586.2021.1994508

The American Professional Society on the Abuse of Children (APSAC). (2012). *Practice guidelines: Forensic interviewing in cases of suspected child abuse.* Author.

The American Professional Society on the Abuse of Children (APSAC). (2016). *APSAC position paper on allegations of child maltreatment and intimate partner violence in divorce/parental relationship dissolution.* http://apsaclibrary.org/positions_all.php#

The American Professional Society on the Abuse of Children (APSAC). (2019). *Practice guidelines: The investigation and determination of suspected psychological maltreatment in children and adolescents.* Author.

Timmons-Mitchell, J., Bender, M. B., Kishna, M. A., & Mitchell, C. C. (2006). An independent effectiveness trial of multisystemic therapy with juvenile justice youth. *Journal of Clinical Child and Adolescent Psychology: The Official Journal for the Society of Clinical Child and Adolescent Psychology, American Psychological Association, Division 53, 35*(2), 227–236. https://doi.org/10.1207/s15374424jccp3502_6

Tomlinson, C. S., Jiang, L. J., & Holtzworth-Munroe, A. (2019). Intimate partner violence and family law: Focus on separating and divorcing parents. In R. Geffner, J. W. White, L. K. Hamberger, A. Rosenbaum, V. Vaughan-Eden, & V. I. Vieth (Eds.) *Handbook of interpersonal violence and abuse across the lifespan*. Springer. https://doi.org/10.1007/978-3-319-62122-7_144-1

Zajac, K., Randall, J., & Swenson, C. C. (2015). Multisystemic therapy for externalizing youth. *Child and Adolescent Psychiatric Clinics of North America, 24*(3), 601–616. https://doi.org/10.1016/j.chc.2015.02.007

Coercion in families and child resistance to contact with a parent after family separation

Kelly M. Champion

ABSTRACT

Family courts face a rare but vexing problem when children angrily refuse contact with a parent after parents separate. In this paper I discuss the associations among child emotional reactivity, child rejection of parent demands, adverse parenting behavior, and coercive control in intimate partner relationships. Decades of clinical and developmental research have explored how adverse parenting behavior and domestic violence impact child development. Children are more likely to have problems with defiance when parents use negative behavior to exert control over vulnerable children. Similarly, childhood exposure to a caregiver who has exerted or does exert coercive control over an intimate partner positively predicts child behavior problems and vulnerability to excessive fear and anger. The paper concludes with a brief discussion of assessing coercion and helping children who reject contact with a parent.

Close to half of the children in the U.S. live with a parent who is separated or divorced from the other parent (Pew Research Center, 2018). When parents separate, divorce, or remarry, children tend to suffer temporary distress. These children are at the same risk for later or chronic emotional, social, and behavioral problems as children living with their married parents (Amato & Anthony, 2014; Teti, 2018).

When children struggle, there are well-established research supported interventions for several of the most common child emotional and behavioral problems. Effective child treatments are based on developmental research and have been shown to predict more symptom relief than other approaches with fewer risk (Weisz et al., 2013). There is no scientific reason to presume that children who live with single, separated, or divorced parents should not be as likely as their peers to benefit from research supported prevention and intervention programs (Champion & Trane, 2020).

Child resistance and defiance

More than half a century of research has been devoted to helping families when children fight parent requests and demands. The applied and basic research show powerful effects of parent attitudes and parenting behaviors. Some children are vulnerable to being trapped in an escalating cycle of coercive behavior with a coercive caregiver. These children and teens are at higher risk to persistently resist adult demands, refuse to adhere to family rules and routines, react with hostility and behave aggressively. Some of these children will have trouble with angry and aggressive reactions to peers and adults outside the home, and legal problems. All are at risk of being physically abused (Dishion et al., 2016; Patterson et al., 2002).

Childhood exposure to coercive control (CC) of an intimate partner or intimate partner violence (IPV) also positively predicts child defiance (Fritz & Roy, 2020; Galano & Graham-Bermann, 2019). Whereas children in the care of safe, secure, and nurturing adults are at lower risk for emotional and behavioral problems. They are less likely to have marked difficulties meeting parental demands and at lower risk of excessive emotional reactions (Turner et al., 2012).

In this paper I argue that coercive adult behavior is fundamental to understanding, preventing, and intervening with children who resist and refuse contact with a parent. The paper begins with a brief review of the almost six decades of clinical and developmental research into Coercive Family Process Theory (CFP) (Patterson et al., 2002). The work has led to widely accepted treatments for children with problems meeting adult demands and displaying hostility toward others. Next, I present research showing a positive association between coercive control of intimate partners and child defiance and child negative emotional reactivity (Fritz & Roy, 2020; Katz, 2016). I briefly discuss research informed treatments that target coercive parenting behavior and help children cope with the negative emotional and behavioral outcomes associated with exposure to adverse adult behavior. I conclude by advocating that reducing coercive parenting and protecting children from high CC adults is in the best interest of children – especially those who resist and refuse contact with a parent.

Coercion

Adverse parenting behavior and child behavior

Parents spend a great deal of time trying to find a way to control the behavior of their developing children – especially early in life. Parents must keep their child safe from danger while the child learns independent skills needed as the child matures. Children are more likely to develop independence when they grow up in homes where the child feels safe, and the parent helps the child to learn to negotiate the challenges of life (Masten & Kalstabakken, 2018; Pinquart, 2017).

Adverse parenting behavior is when parents use threats, excessive withdrawal of attention, or verbal and physical aggression to force a child to comply. Some vulnerable children react to negative parent behavior with escalating displays of anger, aggression, and refusal to comply. Escalating cycles of negative parent and child adverse reactions are the foundation of a CFP (Patterson et al, 2002).

When families are trapped in CFP cycles, children are at risk for disruptive behavior problems. Children with disruptive behavior have problems with other people. Thus, common symptoms of disruptive behavior problems include frequent and intense displays of anger and hostility, age-inappropriate tantrums, deceit, truancy, and *persistent refusal to meet parent demands*. Also, the children in a CFP are at heightened risk for physical abuse. A few of the chldren growing up in CFP cycles will have significant trouble in the future in the community with other people. These children are more likely to be involved later in the criminal justice system (Dishion et al., 2016; Kaminski & Claussen, 2017; Patterson et al., 2002).

Adverse behavior targeting an intimate partner and child behavior

Most people try to influence their intimate partner's behavior. When couples can cope with conflicts without adverse behavior, such as, denigration, verbal and physical attacks, manipulation, or deceit their children are at lower the risk for mental health problems (Galano & Graham-Bermann, 2019; Katz, 2016).

The most serious harm to children happens when a parent uses adverse behavior to show power over the other parent, to force or manipulate the other parent into behavior that is contrary to their own wishes and desires, or to gain control over family resources at the expense of the other parent. This is not about two parents fighting. *Coercive control* describes a pattern of behavior whereby an adult effectively compels, manipulates, threatens or violently forces an intimate partner to behave in a manner that is contrary to the victim's own interests and goals (Hamberger et al., 2017; Hardesty et al., 2015). CC of a partner is the defining concept of intimate partner abuse. CC can happen without physical violence. When threats, deceit, manipulation, and exploitation precedes a partner's fearful compliance and over time the victim further captulates to escalating demands of a coercive partner to avoid panic feelings, there is evidence of CC.

When children experience one parent to physically attack, terrorize, or threaten the other caregiver, the children can reasonably believe that they and their caregiver are in serious danger. Children do not have enough experience to evaluate risk severity. Such traumatic childhood events positively predict child symptoms of post-traumatic stress disorder (PTSD). This puts children at risk for defiant behavior, extreme fear, and hostile reactions. Child PTSD symptoms include disruptive behavior problems, difficulties with emotion regulation and episodes of extreme fear, avoidance, and withdrawal in face of reminders of the trauma (Fritz & Roy, 2020; Jouriles et al., 2018; Rowe & Jouriles, 2019). Effectively understanding the child's problem depends on identifying all past and present threats to a child's psychological safety. A child's intense emotional and behavioral reactions to a parent with a history of adverse behavior may be reasonable reactions to exposure to CC in the past. These facts should not be ignored in conceptualization and treatment planning.

Coercion in parent–child relationships

Coercive Family Process Theory (CFP) is a well-established developmental model of child disruptive behavior problems (e.g., tantrums, hostility, aggression, lying, persistent child resistance to parental demands and refusal to comply) and parent-child relationship problems. Over nearly six decades, researchers have generated a great deal of empirical evidence supporting this theory and demonstrating effective prevention and interventions for child defiance and hostility (Dishion et al., 2016; Patterson et al., 2002).

According to CFP, adverse parent behaviors that target a vulnerable child precede the risk of the child displaying more developmentally inappropriate, frequent and intense disruptive behaviors. Over time, the parent and child become locked in escalating cycles of adverse reactions. These cycles precede pervasive child behavior problems and a severely damaged parent-child relationship. A significant number of children who have been in a CFP will later commit serious moral violation and be involved in the criminal justice system (Dishion et al. 2016).

A CFP starts when a parent uses adverse behavior to try to force a child to comply with directions or follow routines and rules. Adverse parent behaviors include hostile demands for compliance, threats, verbal and physical aggression, guilt induction, manipulation, deceit, shaming, excessive isolation, and repeated humiliation to punish the child. In a CFP, a vulnerable child reacts to adverse parenting behaviors with angry, aggressive resistance. The coercive parent then escalates the adverse behavior. Over the course of repeated and escalating parent-child adverse behavior cycles, a vulnerable child is at higher risk to react to other adults and peers with hostility or aggression. A few of these children will start to use adverse behaviors to meet their own goals. Like the parent who has taught them, these children will use adverse behavior to assert power without provocation. For example, the children will use verbal and physical aggression, manipulation, and threats to dominate and control other children. The child may also lie and cheat to obtain resources and privileges or to retaliate against someone who has injured or threatened the child (Dishion et al., 2016; Patterson, 2002).

Positive parenting behaviors negatively predict disruptive behavior problems. Positive parenting behaviors include frequent praise for specific behavior, emotional sensitivity to the child, and developmentally appropriate supervision. When there is little positive parenting in the home the risk of negative child behavior is higher. Thus, when parents are uninvolved, emotionally insensitive, or inattentive to children, children are at higher risk for disruptive behavior problems, helplessness, and poor social development (Dishion et al., 2016; Masten & Kalstabakken, 2018; Turner et al., 2012).

Treatment and prevention of child resistance to parents

Studies of families in treatment for CFP find that after parents consistently practice positive parenting skills and eliminate adverse parenting behaviors and children are more likely to display fewer disruptive behavior problems (Dishion et al., 2016; Patterson et al., 2002). Studies of children and families around the world, in treatment settings and diverse communities support this theory. Applied research with families show that treatments based on CFP theory are widely accepted as the first line of treatment to reduce the chances that an at-risk child will suffer lasting problems with defiance, tantrums, aggressive behavior, and refusal to comply with parent directions. In families with longstanding CFP, however, parents of teens are at higher risk to be entrenched in frustration with their adolescent and negative expectations of their child. In these families, there is a high risk for the adolescent – parent relationship to be so damaged that treatment must bring in a surrogate adult caregiver. The children are removed from their parents's care. The teens' parents are included in treatment sometimes but only after the parents met specific behavioral treatment goals and demonstrated more positive attitudes and behaviors toward their children (Dishion et al., 2016).

CFP is the theoretical foundation for some of the most widely practiced cognitive-behavioral treatment modules for child and adolescent disruptive behaviors: parent behavior management therapy (Kaminski & Claussen, 2017; Weisz et al. 2013). These treatments are positively associated with more positive parenting behavior, less child disruptive behavior and fewer child emotional problems in many settings including the family court setting (Kaminski & Claussen, 2017; Wolchik, 2013).

Thus, parent-directed treatments for children who have a parent with a history of coercive parenting are the first line of effective treatment for child resistance to parent demands (Dishion et al., 2016; Kaminski & Claussen, 2017; Weisz et al., 2013). When parents increase the frequency of their positive parent behaviors, eliminate harsh or abusive discipline, and consistently practice positive attention, age-appropriate supervision, and emotionally sensitive support toward their child, the parent-child relationship quality is likely to improve as well as the child's adherence to the parent's rules and routines.

Coercive control and intimate partner violence

Whether or not the family is separated, children of all ages in homes with IPV and CC are at higher risk for disruptive behavior problems (Fritz & Roy, 2020; Galano & Graham-Bermann, 2019; Jouriles et al. 2018). Childhood exposure to CC also predicts more cognitive, emotional, and social problems (Fritz & Roy, 2020; Galano & Graham-Bermann, 2019; Rossman, 2001). Exposed children are more likely struggle with rage, fearful avoidance, or a heightened sense of threat. Ordinary developmental challenges can be overwhelming for these children.

Identifying coercive control

Threats and violence in an intimate partner relationship are personal and might be meaningfully threatening only to the victim. How a victim reacts to the adverse behavior, the goals of the perpetrator and the consequences must inform a decision about coercive control and are essential to identifying CC (Hamberger et al., 2017; Katz, 2016). For example, a controlling partner might demand sex from the victim while a young child is sleeping near the couple. The victim may hope the child stays asleep so the victim will minimize displays of fear or protests to try to protect the child. The victim's motivation for complying exposes the abuse and manipulation.

Perpetrators of CC also may make arbitrary demands to demonstrate power (Crossman & Hardesty, 2018; Katz, 2016). For example, a controlling parent might insist that rather than follow routine mealtimes, family members are only permitted to eat when the controlling partner wants to eat. If an abuser locks a family car up at work and traps a victimized parent and children at home, the victim and children are forced to negotiate challenges and possibly deprivation in compliance with an abuser's display of power (Crossman & Hardesty, 2018). Thus, evaluators need more than a frequency count of adverse behaviors by each caregiver to identify a pattern of CC.

Fear that the controlling partner will become violent or more seriously violent often keeps victims from leaving a high CC relationship (Crossman & Hardesty, 2018; Katz, 2016). This fear is realistic. The end of an abusive relationship predicts a higher risk for the victim or her children to be murdered by a former abusive partner (Campbell et al. 2003; Jaffee et al., 2017). Evaluators should consider this factor when accounting for victim's past decisions.

Child adjustment and coercive control

Coercive control directly and indirectly disrupts a victimized parent's caregiving behavior. A controlling partner might limit the victim's freedom of movement and interfere with with a victim's effort to provide for the child's physical, psychological, educational, and social needs. Research suggests that children may suffer more severe social, emotional, and behavior problems from CC when there is a low incidence of severe physical violence. This may be because it is harder for victims to communicate their experience and get protection (Crossman & Hardesty, 2018).

Thus, children in families with a history of IPV or CC also are at a high risk for negative developmental outcomes - even if the child was not present during the IPV. This is because of the victimized parent's efforts to reduce the violence and comply with coercive partner, the victim's high level of stress and fear, and the ways in which the victim complies that may not be responsive to the child's needs (Galano & Graham-Bermann, 2019; Jaffee et al., 2003). The research shows that childhood experiences of CC are positively associated child disrupted behavior problems and child problems with intense negative emotions (e.g., rage, terror, etc.) and emotional reactivity (Crossman & Hardesty, 2018; Fritz & Roy, 2020). It is the same during and after divorce. After separation, the more time a child has in the care of parent with a history of CC, the greater the risk that the child will have behavioral problems (Grasso et al., 2016; Jaffee et al., 2003; Jouriles et al., 2018).

Coercion in families

CFP and CC co-occur. Perpetrators of CC are more likely to engage in adverse parenting behavior and more likely to maltreat a child who is in their care (Fritz & Roy, 2020; Graham-Bermann & Howell, 2011; Grasso et al., 2016). Fathers with a history of CC are less likely to show their children warmth and emotional sensitivity (Stover & Morgos, 2013). Victims of CC are at higher risk for impaired parenting due to the stress of being threatened and manipulated (Galano & Graham-Bermann, 2019). And victimized mothers and children may benefit when provided behavioral management therapy (Wolchik et al., 2013).

Mothers, fathers, children and coercion in families

Fathers are most likely to perpetrate CC of mothers (Hamberger et al., 2017). Men are usually bigger, more powerful and have more access to wealth. While women have more culturally enforced family responsibilities that make it easier for fathers to control mothers (Crossman & Hardesty, 2018; Hamberger et al., 2017).

Less is known about mothers who perpetrate CC against their partners. When women use aggression, they are far less likely to trigger fear in men. Men also rarely change their behavior to accommodate a female partner's demand for control or isolate them from the community according to research (Hamberger et al., 2017). Male victims of violence by female partners report suffering hurt, jealousy, and humiliation but not fear (Hester et al., 2017). Case specific assessments of CC are needed. Evaluators should make clear, behavioral assessments for CC with close attention to the sequence of events and consequences of violence to victims, the children and the family system. A sequential analysis of goals, intentions, and consequences can help evaluators who are confronted with an unusual case presentation such as female perpetrators of CC and IPV.

Conceptualizing family adjustment after separation

Predivorce family characteristics predict the likelihood of child problems after divorce (Peris & Emery, 2004; Polak & Saini, 2019). A parent who has used adverse behavior to gain compliance from any family member is at higher risk to have a poorer parent-child relationship. That fact should inform the assessment and treatment child resistance to parental commands and expectations after family separation. Child refusal to have contact with a parent – especially when the child displays rage, hostility, or fearful withdrawal – is positively predicted from childhood experiences with adverse parent behavior, IPV and CC in the home, and other forms of child maltreatment.

When families come to the family court with children who resist parent directions and refuse to comply with transition, assessment should evaluate parenting history and behavior. Treatments should protect the child from continuing exposure to coercive parenting behavior because protection is effective and in the best interest of child well-being (Kaminski & Claussen, 2017; Kolko et al., 2014). It is not helpful to understanding child behavior if an evaluator diminishes the risks to child adjustment associated with adverse parenting because child protection officials did not find a parent guilty of child abuse (Cross & Hershkowitz, 2017; Saunders, 2015). Adverse parenting behaviors that continue without treatment are likely to worsen over time. Treatment plans that ignore this fact are unlikely to help improve transitions between households.

Caregiver perpetrated trauma also is associated with more problems in the perpetrator parent and child relationship because of the effect of the coercion on the child. Children with PTSD are at risk to react to reminders of their traumatic experiences with escalated and irrational fear – the perpetrating parent may be a reminder. Thus, after a child has exposed to a CFP or CC, the child should be assessed for PTSD. A child's fear, avoidance of and exaggerated hypervigilance might be explained by the child's trauma symptoms. When children grow up with CC, children will often not be able to articulate what triggers their reactions. Expert assessment of child exposure to CC and the child's emotions and behaviors are important to generating an effective plan.

Assessment of parenting behavior

Studies of parent-child relationships and child mental health outcomes show that child reports of parenting quality and emotional connection to a parent strongly predict future outcomes (De Los Reyes et al., 2019; Di Giunta et al., 2020; Jager et al., 2016) Courts should be cautious if an evaluator bases recommendations for families on clinical impressions that diminish reports of coercion and adverse parenting by a child. It is difficult and unreliable moreover to fully assess parenting behavior and identify harmful parents via in-office observations and rating scales (Cross & Hershkowitz, 2017; Saunders et al., 2015). Observational assessments of parents and children are neither complete nor reliable assessments of parenting because these are snapshots of behavior. Parents and children modify their behavior under observation. For example, if children fear punishment out of sight of the observer, a child may modify behavior. The child also may feel safer because they will not be abused in front of an observer. Child interviews and other indirect measures of parenting behavior should be applied.

Treatment of coercion in families

Childhood experiences with coercive parents who target family members predicts more emotional and behavioral problems in children and childhood exposure to IPV, CC or child maltreatment is traumatic. Child victims of trauma are at greater risk for negative emotions and disruptive behavior. Children who do not have any experiences with adverse parent behavior, IPV, CC or CFP are less likely to have persistent problems with refusal to comply with parents regardless of family status.

There are several well-researched and effective treatments for children and teens who resist and refuse parent expectations with hostility or terror. These are well-established evidence-supported mental health interventions (Kaminski & Claussen, 2017). The research shows that parent-child relationships are most likely to improve after parents learn and practice positive parenting. When a parent with a history of harsh or abusive parenting successfully masters these skills and takes responsibility for having threatened or harmed their child, the children also are less likely to be re-victimized (Kolko et al., 2014). Mothers who are the victim of a father's

CC – do not have the power to prevent nor improve father related risks to the father-child relationship (Hamberger et al., 2017). That work rests in fathers' hands (Stover & Morgos, 2013).

Discussion

When children are required to have contact with parents who are or have been emotionally insensitive, inattentive, demanding of child compliance and lacking positive age-appropriate discipline practices, the parent's behavior poses a credible risk to the child's behavioral and emotional well-being (Turner et al., 2012; Zvara et al., 2016). The children who have been exposed a coercive parent are more likely to react to contact with that parent with hostility, to refuse to comply with the demands of that parent, to avoid that parent and to not trust that parent (Dishion et al., 2016).

Parents with a history of perpetrating IPV or CC are at higher risk to abuse or harshly discipline a child and to have few or no positive parenting behaviors. For this reason, there is a higher risk for the child to resist contact with the parent. Only when family court evaluators conduct a detailed assessment of parenting behavior, give close attention to coercion, and include past exposure will the court have enough information to address this risk factor. Court orders that increase a child's time with a parent who is harsh and reduce a child's time with a parent who is safe, secure, and nurturing, risk harm to the child (Jaffee et al., 2003; Turner et al., 2012; Zvara et al., 2016).

Conclusion

Decades of exceptional research have generated well-established science to inform a court officiating over cases with evidence of harsh, emotionally insensitive, abusive and/or coercive parenting. Professionals who advise courts should inform the court of the fact that positive parenting behavior predicts positive parent-child relationships and harsh, insensitive, or abusive parent behavior predicts child behavior and mental health problems.

Incomplete assessments of allegations of coercion may increase the risk of child resistance to transitions after family separation. If the court is unaware of CC and the negative impact of CC on the children, court decisions could require a child to have contact with an untreated or unsuccessfully treated perpetrator of CC. This decision potentially risks more exposures to coercion, increased child resistance to transitions, child resentment and fear.

It is in the best interest of the child when courts are informed of the effects of coercion in families, parent-child relationships, and child behavior. When there is evidence that a parent has used adverse behavior there is a high risk of negative consequences to all family members. The greatest threat is to children.

Disclosure statement

Kelly Champion has no financial or personal interests related to this work.

ORCID

Kelly M. Champion http://orcid.org/0000-0002-6232-4524

References

Amato, P. R., & Anthony, C. J. (2014). Estimating the effects of parental divorce and death with fixed effects models. *Journal of Marriage and the Family*, *76*(2), 370–386. https://doi.org/10.1111/jomf.12100

Campbell, J. C., Webster, D., Koziol-McLain, J., Block, C., Campbell, D., Curry, M. A., Gary, F., Glass, N., McFarlane, J., Sachs, C., Sharps, P., Ulrich, Y., Wilt, S. A., Manganello, J., Xu, X., Schollenberger, J., Frye, V., & Laughon, K. (2003). Risk factors for femicide in abusive relationships: Results from a multisite case control study. *American Journal of Public Health*, *93*(7), 1089–1097. https://doi.org/10.2105/AJPH.93.7.1089

Champion, K. M., & Trane, S. T. (2020). Children of divorce amid allegations of violence need clinical child expertise: Adapting empirically supported interventions. Evidence-Based Practice in *Child and Adolescent Mental Health*, *5*(3), 365–378. https://doi.org/10.1080/23794925.2020.1784059

Cross, T. P., & Hershkowitz, I. (2017). Psychology and child protection: Promoting widespread improvement in practice. *Psychology, Public Policy, and Law*, *23*(4), 503–518. https://doi.org/10.1037/law0000141

Crossman, K., & A., Hardesty, J. (2018). Placing coercive control at the center: What makes coercive control and what makes control coercive. *Psychology of Violence*, *8*(2), 196–206. https://doi.org/10.1037/vio0000094

De Los Reyes, A., Ohannessian, C. M., & Racz, S. J. (2019). Discrepancies between adolescent and parent reports about family relationships. *Child Development Perspectives*, *13*(1), 53–58. https://doi.org/10.1111/cdep.12306

Di Giunta, L., Rothenberg, W. A., Lunetti, C., Lansford, J. E., Pastorelli, C., Eisenberg, N., Thartori, E., Basili, E., Favini, A., Yotanyamaneewong, S., Peña Alampay, L., Al-Hassan, S. M., Bacchini, D., Bornstein, M. H., Chang, L., Deater-Deckard, K., Dodge, K. A., Oburu, P., Skinner, A. T., … Uribe Tirado, L. M. (2020). Longitudinal associations between mothers' and fathers' anger/irritability expressiveness, harsh parenting, and adolescents' socioemotional functioning in nine countries. *Developmental Psychology*, *56*(3), 458–474. https://doi.org/10.1037/dev0000849

Dishion, T., Forgatch, M., Chamberlain, P., & Pelham, W. E. (2016). The Oregon model of behavioral family therapy: From intervention design to promoting large-scale system change. *Behavior Therapy*, *47*(6), 812–837. https://doi.org/10.1016/j.beth.2016.02.002

Fritz, P. A. T., & Roy, E. (2020). Relation between exposure to parental intimate partner violence during childhood and children's functioning. In Geffner R., Vieth V., Vaughan-Eden V., Rosenbaum A., Hamberger L., White J. (eds) *Handbook of interpersonal violence across the lifespan*. Springer. https://doi.org/10.1007/978-3-319-62122-7_312-1

Galano, M. M., & Graham-Bermann, S. A. (2019). Traumatic stress within the family. In B. H. Fiese, M. Celano, K. Deater-Deckard, E. N. Jouriles, & M. A. Wisman (Eds.). *APA handbook of contemporary family psychology: Applications and broad impact of family psychology* (pp. 539–554). American Psychological Association. https://doi.org/10.1037/0000100-033

Graham-Bermann, S. A., & Howell, K. H. (2011). Child maltreatment in the context of intimate partner violence (pp. 167–180). In J. E. B. Myers (Ed.) *The APSAC Handbook on Child Maltreatment* (3rd ed.). Thousand Oaks, CA: Sage Publication, Inc.

Grasso, D. J., Henry, D., Kestler, J., Nieto, R., Wakschlag, L. S., & Briggs-Gowan, M. J. (2016). Harsh parenting as a potential mediator of the association between intimate partner violence and child disruptive behavior in families with young children. *Journal of Interpersonal Violence, 31*(11), 2102–2126. https://doi.org/10.1177/0886260515572472

Hamberger, K. L., Larsen, S. E., & Lehrner, A. (2017). Coercive control in intimate partner violence. *Aggression and Violent Behavior, 37*(1), 1–11. https://doi.org/10.1016/j.avb.2017.08.003

Hardesty, J. L., Crossman, K. A., Haselschwerdt, M. L., Raffaelli, M., Ogolsky, B. G., & Johnson, M. P. (2015). Toward a standard approach to operationalizing coercive control and classifying violence types. *Journal of Marriage and the Family, 77*(4), 833–843. https://doi.org/10.1111/jomf.12201

Hester, M., Jones, C., Williamson, E., Fahmy, E., & Feder, G. (2017). Is it coercive controlling violence? A cross-sectional domestic violence and abuse survey of men attending general practice in England. *Psychology of Violence, 7*(3), 417–427. https://doi.org/10.1037/vio0000107

Jaffee, P., Fairbairn, J., & Reif, K. (2017). Children at risk of homicide in the context of intimate partner violence. In J. C. Campbell & J. T. Messing (Eds.) *Assessing dangerousness: Domestic violence offenders and child abusers* (pp. 179–190). Springer Publishing Company.

Jaffee, S. R., Moffitt, T. E., Caspi, A., & Taylor, A. (2003). Life with (or without) father: The benefits of living with two biological parents depend on the father's antisocial behavior. *Child Development, 74*(1), 109–126. PMID: 12625439. https://doi.org/10.1111/1467-8624.t01-1-00524

Jager, J., Mahler, A., An, D., Putnick, D. L., Bornstein, M. H., Lansford, J. E., Dodge, K. A., Skinner, A. T., & Deater-Deckard, K. (2016). Early adolescents' unique perspectives of maternal and paternal rejection: Examining their across-dyad generalizability and relations with adjustment one year later. *Journal of Youth and Adolescence, 45*(10), 2108–2114. https://doi.org/10.10007/s0964-016-0509z

Jouriles, E. N., Rosenfield, D., McDonald, R., Vu, N. L., Rancher, C., & Mueller, V. (2018). Children exposed to intimate partner violence: conduct problems, interventions, and partner contact with the child. *Journal of Clinical Child and Adolescent Psychology : The Official Journal for the Society of Clinical Child and Adolescent Psychology, American Psychological Association, Division 53, 47*(3), 397–409. https://doi.org/10.1080/15374416.2016.1163706

Kaminski, J. W., & Claussen, A. H. (2017). Evidence base update for psychosocial treatments for disruptive behaviors in children. *Journal of Clinical Child and Adolescent Psychology : The Official Journal for the Society of Clinical Child and Adolescent Psychology, American Psychological Association, Division 53, 46*(4), 477–499. https://doi.org/10.1080/15374416.2017.1310044

Katz, E. (2016). Beyond the physical incident model: how children living with domestic violence are harmed by and resist regimes of coercive control. *Child Abuse Review, 25*(1), 46–59. https://doi.org/10.1002/car.2422

Kolko, D. J., Fitzgerald, M. M., & Laubach, J. L. (2014). Evidence-based practice for working with physically abusive families: Alternatives for families: A cognitive-behavioral therapy. In R. M. Reece, R. F. Hanson & J. Sargent (EDs) *Treatment of child abuse: Common ground for mental health, medical, & legal practitioners*, 2nd ed. (pp. 59–66).

Masten, A. S., & Kalstabakken, A. W. (2018). Developmental perspectives on psychopathology in children and adolescents. In J. N Butcher & P. C. Kendall (Ed.'s) *APA Handbook of Psychopathology*. American Psychological Association. https://doi.org/10.1037/0000065-002

Patterson, G. R., Reid, J. B., & Eddy, J. M. (2002). *A brief history of the Oregon model.* In J. B. Reid, G. R. Patterson, & J. Snyder (Eds.), *Antisocial behavior in children and adolescents: A developmental analysis and model for intervention* (p. 3–20). American Psychological Association. https://doi.org/10.1037/10468-001

Pew Research Center (April (2018). "The Changing Profile of Unmarried Parents." www.pewreseach.org.

Peris, T. S., & Emery, R. E. (2004). A prospective study of the consequences of marital disruption for adolescents: Predisruption family dynamics and postdisruption adolescent adjustment. *Journal of Clinical Child and Adolescent Psychology : The Official Journal for the Society of Clinical Child and Adolescent Psychology, American Psychological Association, Division 53*, *33*(4), 694–704. https://doi.org/10.1207/s15374424jccp3304_5

Pinquart, M. (2017). Associations of parenting dimensions and styles with externalizing problems of children and adolescents: An updated meta-analysis. *Developmental Psychology*, *53*(5), 873–932. https://doi.org/10.1037/dev0000295

Polak, S., & Saini, M. (2019). The complexity of families involved in high-conflict disputes: A postseparation ecological transactional framework. *Journal of Divorce & Remarriage*, *60*(2), 117–140. https://doi.org/10.1080/10502556.2018.1488114

Rossman, R. B. B. (2001). Long term effect of children's exposure to domestic violence. In S. A. Graham-Bermann & J. L. Edleson (Eds.). *Domestic violence in the lives of children: The future of research, intervention, and social policy* (pp. 35–65). American Psychological Association.

Rowe, L. S., & Jouriles, E. N. (2019). Intimate partner violence and the family. In B. H. Fiese, M. Celano, K. Deater-Deckard, E. N. Jouriles, & M. A. Wisman (Eds.). *APA handbook of contemporary family psychology: applications and broad impact of family psychology* (pp. 399–416). American Psychological Association.

Saunders, D. G. (2015). Research based recommendations for child custody evaluation practices and policies in cases of intimate partner violence. *Journal of Child Custody*, *12*(1), 71–92. https://doi.org/10.1080/15379418.2015.1037052

Stover, C. S., & Morgos, D. (2013). Fatherhood and intimate partner violence: Bringing the parenting role into intervention strategies. *Professional Psychology, Research and Practice*, *44*(4), 247–256. /https://doi.org/10.1037/a0031837

Teti, D. M. (2018). Parenting at risk and contemporary family systems. In E.N. Jouriles & M. A. Whisman (Eds.). *APA handbook of contemporary family psychology: foundations, methods, and contemporary issues across the lifespan* (pp. 503–519). American Psychological Association. https://doi.org/10.1037/0000099-028

Turner, H., A., Finkelhor, D., Ormrod, R., Hamby, S., Leeb, R. T., Mercy, J. A., & Holt, M. (2012). Family context, victimization, and child trauma symptoms: Variations in safe, stable, and nurturing relationships during early and middle childhood. *The American Journal of Orthopsychiatry*, *82*(2), 209–219.

Weisz, J. R., Ugueto, A. M., Cheron, D. M., & Herren, J. (2013). Evidence-based youth psychotherapy in the mental health ecosystem. *Journal of Clinical Child and Adolescent Psychology : The Official Journal for the Society of Clinical Child and Adolescent Psychology,*

American Psychological Association, Division 53, 42(2), 274–286. https://doi.org/10.1080/15374416.2013.764824

Wolchik, S. A., Sandler, I. N., Tein, J.-Y., Mahrer, N. E., Millsap, R. E., Winslow, E., Vélez, C., Porter, M. M., Luecken, L. J., & Reed, A. (2013). Fifteen-year follow-up of a randomized trial of a preventive intervention for divorced families: Effects on mental health and substance use outcomes in young adulthood. *Journal of Consulting and Clinical Psychology, 81*(4), 660–673. https://doi.org/10.1037/a0033235

Zvara, B. J., Mills-Koonce, W. R., & Cox, M. (2016). Intimate partner violence, maternal gatekeeping, and child conduct problems. *Family Relations, 65*(5), 647–660. https://doi.org/10.111/fare.12221

"He was the king of the house" children's perspectives on the men who abused their mothers

Simon Lapierre, Isabelle Côté and Geneviève Lessard

ABSTRACT

Children living with domestic violence are exposed to the multiple strategies used by perpetrators to control their mothers, which affects their safety and well-being. However, limited research has investigated children's relationships with their fathers or their mothers' partners in this context. This gap in the literature is problematic, as investigating children's relationships with these men is critical in order to fully understand their experiences and develop policies and practices that respect their rights and adequately respond to their needs. This article reports findings from a study that was conducted with children, and focuses on their relationships with the perpetrators, both before and after separation. The study drew upon a participatory and qualitative methodology, which involved focus groups and individual interviews with 59 participants aged between 6 and 18 years. The research findings revealed that children's relationships with their fathers and mothers' partners had been characterized by violence and control, which had resulted in a range of negative feelings. Several participants reported that they had been relieved to have limited or no contact with these men since separation. While some participants expressed ongoing fear, a few participants noted that the relationships with their fathers had improved during this period.

> We were always at his service. Him, him, him, and him. He only thinks about himself…He was the king of the house. All the time he was pretending to be the king of the house (Research participant, 11-year-old girl).

Children living with domestic violence are exposed to the perpetrators' violent behaviors, and to the multiple strategies they use to control their mothers and other family members (Callaghan et al., 2018; Katz, 2016; Morris, 2009; Øverlien, 2013). They may also observe their mothers' distress or injury, and witness the arrest of either their fathers or their mothers' partners (Mullender et al., 2002). In this context, men's violence creates tensions and fears in their homes, and affects both women's and children's safety and well-being (Katz, 2016; Øverlien, 2013).

Over the last few decades, research on "parenting" in the context of domestic violence has primarily focused on abused women's mothering and mother-child relationships (Arnull & Stewart, 2021; Lapierre, 2008, 2021; Radford & Hester, 2006). This can be explained by the fact that women's mothering and mother-child relationships have been identified as protective factors for children living with domestic violence (Letourneau et al., 2007; Levendosky et al., 2011), and children generally see their mothers as their primary source of protection and support (Lapierre et al., 2018; Mullender et al., 2002). It also reflects the fact that women are still perceived as responsible for ensuring their children's safety and well-being in all circumstances (Krane et al., 2013; Moulding et al., 2015; Wendt et al., 2015).

In contrast, limited research has investigated children's relationships with their fathers or their mothers' partners in the context of domestic violence, particularly from their own perspectives (Holt, 2015; Scott, 2021). This gap in the literature is problematic, as it contributes to shift the focus away from men's violence and therefore reinforces discourses and practices that blame women for "failing to protect" their children (Krane et al., 2013; Lapierre, 2008, 2021; Strega et al., 2003). Moreover, investigating children's relationships with their fathers or their mothers' partners is critical in order to fully understand their experiences and to develop policies and practices that respect their rights and adequately respond to their needs (Lamb et al., 2018). This is particularly relevant to inform decisions in child custody and child protection proceedings (Holt, 2015; Katz et al., 2020; Lamb et al., 2018).

In order to fill this gap in the literature, this article reports findings from a Canadian study that was conducted with children who had experienced domestic violence, focusing on the participants' relationships with their fathers and their mothers' partners. It is divided into four sections, starting with a review of the relevant literature in this area. The following section presents the research objectives, methodology and methods. The third section exposes the research findings, followed by a discussion that addresses implications for policies and practices.

Literature review

Drawing upon research that highlights the connection between domestic violence and child abuse, feminist scholars and activists have challenged the idea that abusive men are "good enough" fathers (Eriksson & Hester,

2001). In the same perspective, Harne (2011) argues that men's violence ought to be taken into account in their fathering:

> Violent fathers' behavior carries over into their parenting and attitudes towardchildren, rather than being a separate issue from violence toward mothers. Because ofthis, their increased involvement in children's care needs to be recognized as puttingchildren at increased risk from abusive parenting practices (p. 179).

However, research evidence shows that many professionals struggle to adequately address the links between domestic violence, men's fathering and father-child relationships in child custody and child protection proceedings (Featherstone & Fraser, 2012; Harne, 2011). On one hand, there is a tendency to focus on abused women's mothering and on their (in) ability to protect their children, while failing to meaningfully engage with men as both perpetrators and fathers (Holt, 2015; Krane et al., 2013; Strega et al., 2003). Featherstone and Peckover (2007) argue that "as part of offering better interventions to women and children, men as fathers need to be engaged with also" (p. 197). On the other hand, the emphasis on fathers' involvement and father-child relationships in child custody proceedings tends to obscure men's violence, particularly post-separation violence, and to minimize its impacts on women's and children's safety and well-being (Harne, 2011; Harrison, 2006; Hester, 2011; Holt, 2015). Even when men's violence has been identified, it is not necessarily seen as a relevant issue in decisions regarding child custody and child contact (Kelly, 2011; Macdonald, 2016). In a Canadian study, Kelly (2011) notes that judges tend to rule on the "maximum contact" principle, and to consider that men's violence toward their partners (children's mothers) should not influence in any way their right to engage with their children. The research findings showed that most fathers had been granted contact, even when the children had witnessed them hitting their mothers or when they had sustained injuries during a violent incident. Kelly (2011) also points out that judges can rule to maintain father-child relationships even when it is contrary to the children's wishes.

Over the last few decades, studies have been conducted with children who have experienced domestic violence, and the research findings provide useful information regarding children's relationships with their fathers and their mother's partners. Overall, those research findings reveal that children living with domestic violence express a range of negative feelings, including fear, confusion, deception, and anger (Buckley et al., 2007; Eskonen, 2005; McGee, 2000; Mullender et al., 2002; Overlien, 2014; Swanston et al., 2014). They tend to express more hostile feelings when they have also been targeted by the perpetrators' violent behaviors (Mullender et al., 2002; Sternberg et al., 2005) and when the perpetrators are not their fathers

(Mullender et al., 2002). In a study conducted by Øverlien and Hydén (2009), one participant mentioned that he had wished someone would have killed his mother's partner, while one participant in Aymer's (2008) study reported that he had attempted to kill his mother's partner. For some children, such actions can be seen as the only way to live free from violence and fear (Øverlien & Hydén, 2009). In contrast, research findings also reveal that some children express that they love their fathers despite their violent behaviors (Aymer, 2008; Dick, 2004; Mullender et al., 2002). While some children side with their fathers (Eisikovits et al., 1998), others hope for change in their fathers' behaviors and want the violence to stop (DeBoard-Lucas & Grych, 2011).

Method

This article reports findings from a study funded by the Canadian Social Sciences and Humanities Research Council (SSHRC), which investigated children's experiences and perspectives on domestic violence in two Canadian provinces: Ontario and Quebec. More specifically, this article focuses on the participants' relationships with the perpetrators, who were either their fathers or their mothers' partners.

Drawing upon a participatory and qualitative methodology, this study gave a voice to children living with domestic violence, valued their perspectives, and fostered their involvement throughout the research process. In the first stage of the study, three focus groups were conducted with 20 children who had experienced domestic violence, in order to initiate a conversation regarding the objectives and modalities of the research. The findings from this first stage were used to ensure that the study focused on issues that were significant to the participants, and to identify the conditions that should be in place in order to collect data in ways that are sensitive to children's needs. They also contributed to the development of a knowledge mobilization strategy.

In the second stage of the study, semi-structured individual interviews were conducted with 46 children who had also experienced domestic violence. These individual interviews, which lasted between 30 and 60 minutes, addressed the following themes: a) their definition and understanding of domestic violence; b) their relationships with their family members; c) their experiences at school and their relationships with their peers; d) their perspectives on social, educational and legal services they had been in contact with. The interview guide had been pre-tested with four children, to ensure that the participants understood the vocabulary used by the researchers. During the interviews, the participants were also invited to draw or create a collage that represented their situation. This facilitated relationship building between the interviewees and the interviewers, and allowed the participants to feel more comfortable during the interviews (see also Harden et al., 2000; Punch, 2002). It also gave the interviewers access to certain issues that might not have been voiced by the participants otherwise.

In total, 59 children took part in this study—36 girls, 21 boys, and two who did not specify their gender identity. The participants were aged between 6 and 18 years at the time of the interviews, with an average age of 11 years old. Amongst the participants, 36 were from Quebec, and 23 were from Ontario, all of whom identified as Francophone. Fifteen participants had a racialized background, and one identified as Indigenous. All the research participants were recruited through domestic violence shelters, community organizations, and child protection agencies.

All the interviews were digitally recorded, transcribed (verbatim) and coded using NVivo 10. The coding tree had eight main categories and several subcategories. The codes were identified based on both the interview guide and the themes that were raised by the participants during the interviews. Three members of the research team (the principal investigator and two research assistants) initially coded the same two interviews, and an agreement was reached for all the codes. All the research assistants involved in the coding process also had to start by coding those two interviews to ensure consistency. The quotes were translated into English for the purpose of this article.

The study was approved by ethics boards in several organizations, including the University of Ottawa (Ontario) and Laval University (Quebec), as well as two child protection agencies. Considering the sensitive topics addressed during the interviews, the participants' safety and well-being were paramount throughout the research process. In this regard, particular attention was given to the issues of informed consent and confidentiality. Consent was required from the participants themselves, and from their mothers. Procedures were in place to report to child protection services situations where children's safety was compromised. All the participants received a compensation ($25) for their involvement in the study.

It is important to highlight two main limitations. First, all the participants were recruited through either domestic violence shelters, community organizations, or child protection agencies. This was not a representative sample, and it should be noted that children who had been in contact with services could be the ones who had been exposed to more severe violence and who had also experienced abuse or neglect. Second, the professionals who recruited the participants may have acted as gatekeepers, recruiting only children who had a better understanding of their situation, had good communication skills, and had more positive perspectives on service providers.

Results

During the individual interviews, the participants described several incidents where their fathers or their mothers' partners had perpetrated violence toward their mothers. Except in one case where it was not possible to identify who the main perpetrator had been, the participants overwhelmingly described situations where the violence had been perpetrated by men. In 30 cases, the main perpetrators had been the participants' fathers, while their mothers' partners had been identified as the main perpetrators in 15 cases.

The research findings presented below reveal that, overall, children's relationships with their fathers and mothers' partners had been characterized by those men's violence and control, which had resulted in a range of negative feelings. The participants also reported post-separation violence and control, and the long-term impacts of these men's behaviors on their safety and well-being. However, the separation had been a significant point in the participants' relationships with their fathers or mothers' partners. While several participants reported that they had had limited or no contact with these men following the separation, a few participants noted that the relationships with their fathers had improved during this period. The research findings also address the complex issue of children's love and attachment to their fathers in this particular context.

Relationships characterized by men's violence and control

The participants talked at length about the violence that had been perpetrated by their fathers or their mothers' partners, and more generally about these men's control over all family members. While most violent behaviors had been perpetrated toward their mothers, the participants also reported incidents where they had been abused and their brothers and sisters had been abused by the perpetrators. The perpetrators' behaviors had included verbal, psychological, and physical assaults, as well as repetitive threats, insults and humiliation, as illustrated in the following quote:

> Screaming, they were screaming a lot. One time … Several times, he sweared at my mother. He sweared at us. He's told me, "You're so stupid". It hurts … For me it meant, "I don't love you anymore" (11-year-oldd girl).

The following quote also illustrates some men's control over all the family members, as this participant explained that he and his mother had been forced to spend most of their time confined to one bedroom:

> Me and my mother we used to live in the bedroom, because my dad was using the rest of the space. When we needed to use the washroom or to eat, it was the only times we felt like leaving the bedroom (7-year-old boy).

Several participants explained that the violence and control had continued after the separation. They reported numerous incidents of post-separation violence, some of which had happened during father-child contact arrangements. In the following quote, the respondent mentioned that she had serious doubts regarding her father's willingness or ability to change, leading her to think that her father's violence would never stop:

> My father will never let go until he gets what he wants. That means he will continue until he'll see us weak or sad. I don't know...I don't even know what he wants because he doesn't have custody of the children, and he doesn't have to pay for child support (16-year-old girl).

These men's violence and control had been central and enduring features in the participants' relationships with their fathers or their mothers' partners. They had resulted in a range of negative feelings, which had influenced how they perceived those men and their relationships with them.

Negative feelings resulting from men's violence and control

The participants expressed a range of negative feelings when they talked about their relationships with their fathers or their mothers' partners. Fear was an important theme emerging from the data. Indeed, several respondents reported that they had experienced fear, sometimes intense fear over an extended period of time. In the following quote, one 10-year-old girl explained why she had been scared of her father:

> I'm scared he hits me or something like that, because when we say or do something that is not okay, he... His look, it's scary. I don't know why, but I've always been scared of him (10-year-old girl).

Some participants mentioned that they were still scared of the perpetrators at the time of the interviews, as illustrated in this girl's account:

> I'm still scared because my dad knows where we live. I don't know how he found out. He probably followed us. (...) Sometimes, my mother's car starts beeping and my mother is always scared that it might be him (16-year-old girl).

Several participants also expressed sadness and anger toward their fathers or their mothers' partners. Moreover, some participants stated explicitly that they "hated" those men for what they had done to them and to their mothers, as illustrated in the following quote:

> Right now, I hate my father for many reasons. Because of him, I was exposed to this violence he used towards my mother. He also used violence towards my brothers and myself (14-year-old girl).

While the participants' relationships with their fathers and their mothers' partners had been characterized by these men's violence and control, which had resulted in a range of negative feelings toward them, some participants still expressed love and attachment for their fathers. In contrast, no participant expressed such positive feelings in relation to their mothers' partners. In fact, several children mentioned that they had never trusted their mothers' partners, and that these men had never been significant individuals in their lives. Those respondents explained that, as a result, they had never made any efforts to build meaningful relationships with those men, as illustrated in the following quote:

> I wasn't close to my mother's partner. I saw him and I just felt like puking. I couldn't stand him. Even when I was young, I couldn't stand him (8-year-old girl).

In this context, it is probably not surprising that most respondents had had limited or no contact with their fathers or their mothers' partners following the separation, and that this was generally seen as a positive outcome, even though a few respondents had noted an improvement in their relationships with their fathers during this period.

Limited contact in the post-separation period

At the time of the interviews, most participants had limited or no contact with their fathers or their mothers' partners, and this was generally seen as a positive outcome with regard to their safety and well-being. In this regard, several participants explained that they had felt relieved once they no longer had to see the perpetrators. One 11-year-old girl stated: "When we stopped seeing my father, well it was better" (11-year-old girl).

This was true when the perpetrators had been their fathers, but it was particularly evident when the perpetrators were not their fathers. As mentioned above, several respondents explained that their mothers' partners had never been significant individuals in their lives, and that they had made no efforts to build meaningful relationships with them. Therefore, no participant had wished to have contact with their mothers' partners following the separation. In the following quote, one participant explained how she had felt about her mother's partner leaving their home: "Like I didn't have a good relationship with him, it was just my mother's boyfriend. I was just eager for him to leave our home" (girl, age unknown).

Several children were also happy to have limited or no contact with their fathers, and had not wished to have more contact with them. This was due to their fathers' behaviors and to the violence that they had experienced in the past. They also feared more violent incidents in the future, as they expressed serious doubts regarding their fathers' willingness or ability to change. In fact, some participants reported incidents that had taken place during contact arrangements, and one 8-year-old boy recalled: "We used to have contact with my father, but then it stopped... Because we were scared of him" (8-year-old boy).

While a few participants would have liked to have more frequent contact with their fathers, they realized that having limited or no contact had been a safer and more positive outcome given their fathers' violent behaviors. One 10-year-old girl stated: "It's been a year since I have seen him. But sometimes, he gets really mad and I don't like that... I'd like to see him, but it's his behaviors that scare me" (10-year-old girl). Another participant explained:

> Sometimes I want to see him and sometimes I don't, but I know that it is for the best. It's best that I don't see him because as long as he doesn't want to change, to be less violent and to see a psychologist... He will probably still be mad and I will still be scared (14-year-old girl).

Improving relationships in the post-separation period

A few participants mentioned that their relationships with their fathers had improved during the post-separation period. Such improvements had resulted from positive changes in their fathers' behaviors, including their parenting behaviors. For instance, this respondent explained that her father had been more available in the period following the separation, and had paid more attention to her needs and to her brother's needs:

> At this point my father does more activities with us, you know, we go out more, with him and my brother. Before he wasn't doing much with us. When we would talk to him, he would barely reply to us (12-year-old girl).

However, it should be noted that the children who reported improvements in the relationships with their fathers had not lived with them. In many cases, they had not had contact with them on a daily or even on a regular basis and, according to these participants, such positive changes would not have been possible otherwise. For instance, this 9-year-old girl had had contact with her father, but she did not think it would be safe to live with him: "Now, our father doesn't hit us anymore... Now that he doesn't live with us. Because if he was still living with us, he would still hit us" (9-year-old girl).

The participants who noted improvements in their relationships with their fathers, just like the ones who had had limited or no contact with them, all expressed concerns regarding their mothers' and their own safety and well-being during the post-separation period.

Love and attachment despite the fathers' violence and control

As mentioned above, a few participants expressed love and attachment for their fathers, despite their violent behaviors and control strategies. However, it was very clear in those children's accounts that such feelings had not made their fathers' violence any less visible or problematic. The same participants could express both positive and negative feelings toward their fathers.

Although those appeared to be the participants' genuine feelings toward their fathers, their accounts raise a number of questions. For some respondents, those positive feelings seemed to be rooted in an idealized vision of father-child relationships rather than in positive experiences and memories. In this perspective, children's love and attachment for their fathers seem to be largely taken-for-granted, automatic and unconditional. This 11-year-old girl, who also mentioned at another point during the interview that she hated her father, seemed to draw upon the notion of "unconditional love" in the following quote:

> Yes, I see him, and will continue to see him. Because maybe he doesn't love me, but I still love him… For example, if your father was a murderer, you would still love him. Usually it's like this, for most people. But I'm starting to love him less (11-year-old girl).

In the following quote, one participant also seemed to talk about an "unbreakable connection" between children and their fathers, regardless of the fathers' behaviors: "Even though he hurt us, he will always be my father" (16-year-old girl).

Although those research findings reflect an idealized vision of father-child relationships, it does not mean that these participants idealized their fathers. They were still fully aware of their fathers' violence and control, and recognized the risk for their mothers' and their own safety and well-being.

Discussion

This article reported findings from a study that investigated children's experiences and perspectives on domestic violence, which recognized children as social actors who have their own understandings and their own strategies. More specifically, the research findings presented above focused on children's relationships with their fathers or their mothers' partners. As mentioned above, investigating those children's perspectives on their relationships with those men is critical in order to better understand their experiences, and to develop policies and practices that respect their rights and adequately respond to their needs.

The research findings reveal that, overall, the participants' relationships with their fathers or their mothers' partners had been characterized by those men's violence and control, which had resulted in a range of negative feelings. Findings demonstrate that children recognize men's violent behaviors—including psychological, verbal, and physical assaults—as well as their various control strategies, which can often manifest in more subtle ways. Therefore, children's experiences and relationships with their fathers or their mothers' partners cannot be understood through an incident-based model of domestic violence (Callaghan et al., 2018; Katz, 2016; Morris, 2009; Øverlien, 2013; Stark, 2007). We argue that professionals should not limit their evaluations to specific incidents, and need to take more subtle control strategies into account. Listening to women and children is the best way to understand those control strategies, and how they impact their daily lives. Professionals working with children who have experienced domestic violence also need to engage more significantly with the perpetrators' behaviors, and recognize their impacts on both women's and children's safety and well-being (Featherstone & Peckover, 2007; Harne, 2011; Holt, 2015; Katz et al., 2020). As pointed out by Featherstone and Peckover (2007), "safety planning for women and children must include work with men and work with men must include safety planning for women and children" (p. 197).

The negative feelings that were reported by the participants are consistent with findings from previous studies (Buckley et al., 2007; Eskonen, 2005; McGee, 2000; Overlien, 2014; Øverlien & Hydén, 2009; Swanston et al., 2014). Those negative feelings included fear, sadness and anger, and some participants stated that they "hated" their fathers or their mothers' partners. We argue that professionals working with children who have experienced domestic violence need to validate these feelings as "normal" and "acceptable" in such circumstances. It is important to avoid a pathological lens to look at children's reactions, which constructs children who express anger as having "anger management" or "emotion regulation" problems, or as reproducing the perpetrators' violent attitudes and behaviors. Expression of anger can be seen as a normal response to violence as well as a manifestation of resistance to men's violence and control. We argue that professionals should listen to children who state that they "hate" their fathers instead of interpreting it as a reflection of their mothers' attitudes toward their partners or ex-partners, as noted in the recent literature on parental alienation (Lapierre et al., 2020; Meier, 2009).

While the research findings show that, overall, the participants' relationships with the perpetrators had been characterized by those men's violence and control, and had resulted in a range of negative feelings, they also reveal that children's relationships with their fathers tend to be more complex than the relationships with their mothers' partners. In this regard, a few participants expressed both negative and positive feelings toward their fathers, which was not the case for their mothers' partners. While previous studies have reported children's mixed feelings toward their fathers (Mullender et al., 2002; Ornduff & Monahan, 1999; Peled, 2000), the research findings raise a number of issues that would warrant further investigation. As mentioned above, the participants' accounts suggest that positive feelings such as love and attachment were rooted in an idealized vision of father-child relationships rather than in positive experiences and memories. We argue that professionals should not question whether these are genuine feelings, but they could work with children to unpack their expressions of love and attachment for their fathers, and to reflect on what love and attachment mean to them.

It was clear in the participants' accounts that the positive feelings toward their fathers had not made their violence and control any less visible or problematic. The positive feelings do not replace the negative ones, including fear and anger. Professionals ought to realize that even when children say that they love their fathers or that they would like to spend more time with them, it does not mean that they feel safe and that they want immediate contact. A thorough assessment of these situations still need be conducted, and both women's and children's immediate safety and well-being should be paramount in decisions regarding child custody and child contact.

The research findings highlight particular issues emerging during the post-separation period, which have important implications for child custody and child contact decisions. Children felt relief to be safe and no longer in need of hypervigilance in an attempt to protect themselves and their mothers. Similar issues have been reported in previous studies that have been conducted with adults (Holt, 2015; Lapierre, 2010; Radford & Hester, 2006). First, professionals ought to acknowledge post-separation violence, which include both violent behaviors and a range of control strategies. Their assessments need to recognize the connections between the past and the current situations, between women's and children's victimizations, as well as between women's and children's safety and well-being. We also argue that professionals must create safe spaces where children can express their feelings and wishes, and take them into account in their decisions or recommendations. Children should not be sent to be with a parent they fear will be physically or emotionally abusive to them. Should a violent parent be successful in learning new skills, then gradually lengthening visits with safeguards to protect children might become appropriate if the children desire it.

Given that the participants had not seen their mothers' partners as significant individuals in their lives, and that they had made no efforts to build meaningful relationships with them, the research findings suggest that there should be no efforts to maintain children's relationships with those men following the separation. Regarding children's relationships with their fathers following the separation, several participants had felt relieved to have limited or no contact with them during this period, and had not wished to have more contact with them in the near future. In contrast, a few participants had noted improvements in the relationships with their fathers during this period, but those participants had not lived with them and had not had contact with them on a daily or even on a regular basis. Those research findings challenge the idea that children always want to see their fathers, or that children need fathers who do not employ positive parenting practices. Professionals working with children who have experienced domestic violence need to understand that there are different ways to engage with the perpetrators, and that it does not mean promoting father involvement and father-child relationships when positive and healthy relationships have not been demonstrated in the past. As mentioned above, they should first engage with those men's behaviors to assess both women's and children's safety and well-being, and work toward accountability (Bancroft et al., 2012; Featherstone & Peckover, 2007; Harne, 2011; Holt, 2015; Katz et al., 2020). In this regard, Holt (2015) rightly points out that we need to prioritize "the construction of fathers as 'risk' in the context of post-separation father-child contact" (p. 210). This does not mean that children should never see their fathers, but when children want to see their fathers there should be effective measures in place to ensure their own and their mothers' safety and well-being. However, we argue that father-child relationships should not be maintained at all costs, and that children who have experienced domestic violence should not be forced to see their fathers against their will when they fear for their emotional and physical safety as they grow and develop.

Conclusion

This article has focused on children's relationships with their fathers and their mothers' partners in the context of domestic violence. While most studies on "parenting" in the context of domestic violence have focused on abused women's mothering and mother-child relationships, it is essential to better understand children's relationships with their fathers or their mothers' partners. Children's perspectives should inform policies and practices in this area, because decisions custody and contact can have serious impacts on their safety and well-being. Relationships with individuals who create unsafe emotional and physical environments do not promote healthy development in children.

Disclosure statement

The authors report no conflicts of interest. The authors alone are responsible for the content and writing of the paper.

Ethical standards and informed consent

All procedures followed were in accordance with the ethical standards of the Research Ethics Board at the University of Ottawa, and with the Helsinki Declaration of 1975, as revised in 2000. Informed consent was obtained from all patients for being included in the study.

Funding

The study was supported by a grant from the Canadian Social Sciences and Humanities Research Council (SSHRC).

References

Arnull, E., & Stewart, S. (2021). Developing a theoretical framework to discuss mothers experiencing domestic violence and being subject to interventions: A cross-national perspective. *International Journal for Crime, Justice and Social Democracy, 10*(2), 113–126. https://doi.org/10.5204/ijcjsd.1561

Aymer, S. R. (2008). Adolescent males' coping responses to domestic violence: A qualitative study. *Children and Youth Services Review, 30*(6), 654–664. https://doi.org/10.1016/j.childyouth.2008.01.011

Bancroft, L., Silverman, J. G., & Ritchie, D. (2012). *The batterer as parent: Addressing the impact of domestic violence on family dynamics* (2nd ed.). Sage.

Buckley, H., Whelan, S., & Holt, S. (2007). Listen to me! Children's experiences of domestic violence. *Child Abuse Review, 16*(5), 296–310. https://doi.org/10.1002/car.995

Callaghan, J. E. M., Alexander, J. H., Sixsmith, J., & Fellin, L. C. (2018). Beyond "witnessing": Children's experiences of coercive control in domestic violence and abuse. *Journal of Interpersonal Violence, 33*(10), 1551–1581. https://doi.org/10.1177/0886260515618946

DeBoard-Lucas, R., & Grych, J. (2011). Children's perceptions of intimate partner violence: Causes, consequences, and coping. *Journal of Family Violence, 26*(5), 343–354. https://doi.org/10.1007/s10896-011-9368-2

Dick, G. (2004). Men's relationships with their fathers: Comparing men who batter women with non-violent men. *Journal of Emotional Abuse, 4*(1), 61–84. https://doi.org/10.1300/J135v04n01_04

Eisikovits, Z., Winstok, Z., & Enosh, G. (1998). Children's experience of interparental violence: A heuristic model. *Children and Youth Services Review, 20*(6), 547–568. https://doi.org/10.1016/S0190-7409(98)00025-5

Eriksson, M., & Hester, M. (2001). Violent men as good-enough fathers?: A look at England and Sweden. *Violence Against Women, 7*(7), 779–798. https://doi.org/10.1177/10778010122182730

Eskonen, I. (2005). Violence in children's narration. *International Journal of Child & Family Welfare, 8*(1), 32–45.

Featherstone, B., & Fraser, C. (2012). Working with fathers around domestic violence: Contemporary debates. *Child Abuse Review, 21*(4), 255–263. https://doi.org/10.1002/car.2221

Featherstone, B., & Peckover, S. (2007). Letting them get away with it: Fathers, domestic violence and child welfare. *Critical Social Policy, 27*(2), 181–202. https://doi.org/10.1177/0261018306075708

Harden, J., Scott, S., Backett-Milburn, K., & Jackson, S. (2000). Can't talk, Won't talk: Methodological issues in researching children. *Sociological Research Online, 5*(2), 104–115. https://doi.org/10.5153/sro.486

Harne, L. (2011). *Violent fathering and the risks to children the need for change*. Policy Press.

Harrison, C. (2006). Dammed if you do and dammed if you don't? The contradictions between private and public law. In C. Humphreys & N. Stanley (Eds.), *Domestic violence and child protection: Directions for good practice* (pp. 137–154). Jessica Kingsley.

Hester, M. (2011). The three planets model: Towards an understanding of contradictions in approaches to women and children's safety in contexts of domestic violence. *British Journal of Social Work, 41*(5), 837–853. https://doi.org/10.1093/bjsw/bcr095

Holt, S. (2015). Post-separation fathering and domestic abuse: Challenges and contradictions. *Child Abuse Review, 24*(3), 210–222. https://doi.org/10.1002/car.2264

Katz, E. (2016). Beyond the physical incident model: How children living with domestic violence are harmed by and resist regimes of coercive control. *Child Abuse Review, 25*(1), 46–59. https://doi.org/10.1002/car.2422

Katz, E., Nikupeteri, A., & Laitinen, M. (2020). When coercive control continues to harm children: Post-separation fathering, stalking and domestic violence. *Child Abuse Review, 29*(4), 310–324. https://doi.org/10.1002/car.2611

Kelly, F. (2011). Enforcing a parent/child relationship at all cost? Supervised access orders in the Canadian courts. *Osgoode Hall Law Journal, 49*(2), 277–309.

Krane, J., Strega, S., & Carlton, R. (2013). G-d couldn't be everywhere so he created mothers": The impossible mandate of maternal protection in child welfare. In S. Strega, J. Krane, S. Lapierre, C. Richardson, & R. Carlton (Eds.). *Failure to protect: Moving beyond gendered responses*. Fernwood.

Lamb, K., Humphreys, C., & Hegarty, K. (2018). Your behaviour has consequences": Children and young people's perspectives on reparation with their fathers after domestic violence. *Children and Youth Services Review, 88*, 164–168. https://doi.org/10.1016/j.childyouth.2018.03.013

Lapierre, S. (2008). Mothering in the context of domestic violence: The pervasiveness of a deficit model of mothering. *Child & Family Social Work, 13*(4), 454–463. https://doi.org/10.1111/j.1365-2206.2008.00563.x

Lapierre, S. (2010). Are abused women 'neglectful' mothers? A critical reflection based on women's experiences. In B. Featherstone, C. A. Hooper, J. Scourfield, & J. Taylor (Eds.), *Gender and child welfare in society* (pp. 121–148). Wiley.

Lapierre, S. (2021). Mothering in the context of domesic violence. In Devaney (Eds.), *Routledge international handbook on domestic violence and abuse*. Routledge.
Lapierre, S., Côté, I., Lambert, A., Buetti, D., Lavergne, C., Damant, D., & Couturier, V. (2018). Difficult but close relationships: Children's perspectives on relationships with their mothers in the context of domestic violence. *Violence against Women, 24*(9), 1023–1038.
Lapierre, S., Ladouceur, P., Frenette, M., & Côté, I. (2020). The legitimization and institutionalization of 'parental alienation' in the province of Quebec. *Journal of Social Welfare and Family Law, 42*(1), 30–44. https://doi.org/10.1080/09649069.2019.1701922
Letourneau, N., Fedick, L., & Willms, C. (2007). Mothering and domestic violence: A longitudinal analysis. *Journal of Family Violence, 22*(8), 649–659. https://doi.org/10.1007/s10896-007-9099-6
Levendosky, A., Bogat, G., Huth-Bocks, A., Rosenblum, K., & Von Eye, A. (2011). The effects of domestic violence on the stability of attachment from infancy to preschool. *Journal of Clinical Child and Adolescent Psychology: The Official Journal for the Society of Clinical Child and Adolescent Psychology, American Psychological Association, Division 53, 40*(3), 398–410. https://doi.org/10.1080/15374416.2011.563460
Macdonald, G. S. (2016). Domestic violence and private family court proceedings: Promoting child welfare or promoting contact? *Violence against Women, 22*(7), 832–852. https://doi.org/10.1177/1077801215612600
McGee, C. (2000). *Childhood experiences of domestic violence*. Jessica Kingsley Publishers.
Meier, J. (2009). A historical perspective on parental alienation syndrome and parental alienation. *Journal of Child Custody, 6*(3–4), 232–234. https://doi.org/10.1080/15379410903084681
Morris, A. (2009). Gendered dynamics of abuse and violence in families: Considering the abusive household gender regime. *Child Abuse Review, 18*(6), 414–427. https://doi.org/10.1002/car.1098
Moulding, N. T., Buchanan, F., & Wendt, S. (2015). Untangling self-blame and mother-blame in women's and children's perspectives on maternal protectiveness in domestic violence: Implications for practice. *Child Abuse Review, 24*(4), 249–260. https://doi.org/10.1002/car.2389
Mullender, A., Hague, G., Imam, U., Kelly, L., Malos, E., & Regan, L. (2002). *Children's perspectives on domestic violence*. Sage Publication.
Ornduff, S. R., & Monahan, K. (1999). Children's understanding of parental violence. *Child and Youth Care Forum, 28*(5), 351–364. https://doi.org/10.1023/A:1021974429983
Øverlien, C. (2013). The children of patriarchal terrorism. *Journal of Family Violence, 28*(3), 277–287. https://doi.org/10.1007/s10896-013-9498-9
Øverlien, C., & Hydén, M. (2009). Children's actions when experiencing domestic violence. *Childhood, 16*(4), 479–496. https://doi.org/10.1177/0907568209343757
Overlien, C. (2014). He didn't mean to hit mom, I think': Positioning, agency and point in adolescents' narratives about domestic violence. *Child and Family Social Work, 19*, 156–164.
Peled, E. (2000). The parenting of men who abuse women: Issues and dilemmas. *British Journal of Social Work, 30*(1), 25–36. https://doi.org/10.1093/bjsw/30.1.25
Punch, S. (2002). Research with children: The same of different from research with adults? *Childhood, 9*(3), 321–341. https://doi.org/10.1177/0907568202009003005
Radford, L., & Hester, M. (2006). *Mothering through domestic violence*. Jessica Kingsley Publishers.
Scott. (2021). Fathering in the context of domestic violence and abuse. In Devaney (Eds.), *Routledge international handbook on domestic violence and abuse*. Routledge.

Sternberg, K. J., Lamb, M. E., Guterman, E., Abbott, C. B., & Dawud-Noursi, S. (2005). Adolescents' perceptions of attachments to their mothers and fathers in families with histories of domestic violence: A longitudinal perspective. *Child Abuse & Neglect*, *29*(8), 853–869.

Strega, S., Callahan, M., Rutman, D., & Dominelli, L. (2003). Undeserving mothers: social policy and disadvantaged mothers. *Canadian Review of Social Policy*, *49–50*, 175–198.

Swanston, J., Bowyer, L., & Vetere, A. (2014). Towards a richer understanding of school-age children's experiences of domestic violence: The voices of children and their mothers. *Clinical Child Psychology and Psychiatry*, *19*(2), 184–201. https://doi.org/10.1177/1359104513485082

Wendt, S., Buchanan, F., & Moulding, N. (2015). Mothering and domestic violence: Situating maternal protectiveness in gender. *Affilia: Journal of Women and Social Work*, *30*(4), 533–545. https://doi.org/10.1177/0886109915570925

Examining associations between psychological control and proactive and reactive aggression among middle school age youth

Paula J. Fite, Kathleen I. Díaz and Madelaine R. Abel

ABSTRACT

Parental psychological control has been linked to aggression, but further research is needed to elucidate specific associations with the functions of aggression. The current study sought to advance the field by examining associations between parental psychological control and reactive and proactive aggression and whether symptoms of anxiety moderated these links in a sample of middle school age youth. Youth (N = 290, 50% male and 50% female) completed self-reported measures at school. Findings indicated that while parental psychological control was linked to both reactive and proactive aggression, the link with reactive aggression was most robust. Further, anxiety symptoms were not found to moderate these associations. Results suggest that parental psychological control is linked to aggressive behavior among middle school age youth, particularly for reactive aggression, and these effects are independent of levels of anxiety symptoms.

Growing evidence suggests that parental psychological control (i.e., emotional manipulation of children using guilt and love withdrawal) contributes to aggression, particularly relational aggression (Kuppens et al., 2013). Further knowledge of these links would be helpful for understanding the etiology of aggression, ultimately informing prevention and intervention efforts. However, more research is needed to evaluate the influence of psychological control on the functions of aggression, namely proactive and reactive aggression (McClain et al., 2020), and to evaluate factors that contribute to these associations. One factor to consider is levels of anxiety symptoms, as anxiety may impact youth behavioral responses to parenting tactics, including parental psychological control. The current study examines the role of anxiety symptoms in the links between parental psychological control and proactive and reactive aggression in a sample of middle school age youth.

The two established functions of aggression, reactive and proactive, are distinguished by the intended motivation of the aggressive behavior (Card & Little, 2006; Dodge & Coie, 1987). Proactive aggression is planned, goal-directed, and typically used to achieve a specific goal or reward (Dodge & Coie, 1987). This function of aggression is best understood according to the social learning theory (Bandura, 1973), which states that individuals learn from others modeling and personally experiencing that aggressive behavior generates rewards or adaptive outcomes. That is, youth learn that aggression can help one achieve desired goals and objects by observing others obtain their goals with the use of aggression. Consistent with social learning theory, having parents who engage in aggressive behavior and affiliating with aggressive peers is associated with elevated levels of proactive aggression (Fite et al., 2016; Vitaro et al., 2006).

In contrast, reactive aggression is impulsive or retaliatory behavior that is often enacted in response to perceived threat or frustration (Dodge & Coie, 1987). According to the frustration-anger theory of aggression (Berkowitz, 1993), this type of aggression is an emotional, reactionary response to perceived threat or barriers to gaining rewards. Reactive aggression may develop through inaccurate social information processing, in which youth attribute hostile intent to ambiguous situations and then react aggressively (e.g., child thinks peer bumped into them on purpose and then push the peer; Dodge & Coie, 1987). As such, some etiological risk factors for reactive aggression include inconsistent or unstable environments (e.g., inconsistent parenting), experiencing negative life events (e.g., maltreatment, parent marital conflict), and poor emotion regulation and hyperarousal (e.g., Lamarche et al., 2007; Vitaro et al., 2002; 2006).

Consistent with various theories, such as stress and coping theory (Folkman & Lazarus, 1984) and socio-ecological theory (Bronfenbrenner, 1977), one's parents can influence coping and functioning. Emotionally manipulating children using guilt induction or excessive personal control for parents' own gains are the hallmark characteristics of parental psychological control (Barber, 1996). The mixed emotional responding as well as the modeling of negative responses to behavior associated with psychological control likely results in negative adjustment outcomes, with this parenting approach associated with both internalizing and externalizing problem behaviors (Barber & Harmon, 2002; Kuppens et al., 2013; Loukas et al., 2005; Pinquart, 2017a, 2017b). For example, parental psychological control has been linked to symptoms of anxiety among youth (e.g., Nanda et al., 2012). Moreover, parental psychological control has been broadly linked to aggression (e.g., Loukas et al., 2005), but the most robust link appears to be with relational forms of aggression (i.e., behavior that threatens to damage social relationships; for a meta-analysis see

Kuppens et al., 2013). However, very little research has examined the links between parental psychological control and the functions of aggression.

There is reason to believe that parental psychological control may be linked to both functions of aggression. To date, only limited research has examined associations between parental psychological control and these functions of aggression. One study found that parental psychological control was positively associated with youth self-reports of reactive, but not proactive, aggression among 8-to-12-year-old youths (McClain et al., 2020). In another study of 9-to-12-year-old children, youth-reported psychological control was positively correlated with both teacher-reported proactive and reactive aggression (Rathert et al., 2011). However, psychological control did not predict reactive aggression after controlling for proactive aggression (Rathert et al., 2011). These preliminary studies suggest that there may be differential associations between psychological control and the two distinct functions of aggression, but results may depend on informant. Further, it is not clear under what conditions these associations are most evident.

Anxiety symptoms may be a factor to consider in these links, as anxiety and aggression commonly co-occur (Granic, 2014). More specifically, the literature has consistently found an association between reactive aggression and anxiety symptoms (Card & Little, 2006; Vitaro et al., 2002). This specific link to reactive aggression is likely bidirectional in nature. That is anxiety may make youth hyper-aroused to punishment, resulting in retaliatory reactive aggression, and in turn, reactive aggression may result in anxiety as a result of feeling guilty for overreacting aggressively (Fite et al., 2016). Moreover, anxiety symptoms may moderate the associations between parental psychological control and these functions of aggression. The hyper-arousal effect of anxiety combined with psychological control may result in elevated reactive aggression. In contrast, proactive aggression is associated with low arousal and cold-blooded in nature (e.g., Dodge & Coie, 1987; Fite et al., 2016). Thus, parental psychological control may be more likely to result in proactive aggression when levels of anxiety are low. Indeed, in a sample of emerging adults, Wagner and Abaied (2016) found evidence for the moderating effects of anxiety in the associations between psychological control and reactive and proactive relational aggression. Specifically, they found that parental psychological control was associated with reactive [relational] aggression at high levels of skin conductance reactivity (which is conceptualized as a physiological marker of anxiety within the sympathetic nervous system), whereas parental psychological control was only associated with proactive [relational] aggression at low levels of skin conductance reactivity (which is conceptualized as a physiological marker of low levels of anxiety). However, more research is needed to further evaluate these associations before conclusions can be drawn. The current study examined anxiety symptoms as a moderator of the links between psychological control and proactive and reactive aggression. It was posited that parental psychological control would be most strongly linked to reactive aggression at high levels of anxiety and most strongly linked to proactive aggression at low levels of anxiety.

The current study extends the literature by further examining links between youth reports of parental psychological control and the functions of aggression as youth are transitioning into adolescence, a time of heightened social and emotional challenges and heightened reactivity to interpersonal stress (Hankin et al., 2010; Rudolph & Hammen, 1999). Early adolescence is also a period of increased autonomy development and thus parent psychological control may be particularly problematic during this time (Wagner & Abaied, 2016). It was expected that psychological control would be positively linked to both reactive and proactive aggression, but the link with reactive aggression would be stronger (McClain et al., 2020). Additionally, it was posited that anxiety symptoms would moderate these associations, but the moderating effects would vary based on the function of aggression. Specifically, it was expected that psychological control would be most strongly linked to reactive aggression when levels of anxiety symptoms were high and most strongly linked to proactive aggression when levels of anxiety symptoms were low.

Method

Participants

Participants included 6th (n = 91), 7th (n = 114), and 8th (n = 85) graders from a small rural middle school located in the Midwest area of the United States. From the total 290 participants, six youths did not report on their gender and four youths identified their gender as "other;" these participants were excluded from regression analyses given the inability to control for gender effects in analyses for these youth. Accordingly, 290 youth were included in correlation analyses and 280 youth were included in aggression analyses. Of the participants who identified their gender, 50% identified as male and 50% identified as female, with youths' ages ranging from 11 to 14 (M age = 3.29, SD = .92). The school's administrators provided limited demographics information on the sample; however, consistent with the location of the school, participants predominately identified as White and non-Hispanic.

Procedures

The current study was approved by the researchers' Institutional Review Board as well as the administrators of the middle school prior to data collection. To participate in the study, a legal guardian/parent of each student provided consent. Of the entire student body, 77.36% of students had parental consent to participate in the study (i.e., 311 out of 402 students had parental consent). 290 of these youth with parental permission actually completed the survey, with current data representing 72.14% of the school. On the day of data collection, during the Fall semester of 2018, students who had consent were asked to also give their assent to complete the study. Participants completed a 30-minute confidential online Qualtrics survey, which included self-reporting their age, grade, gender, and a battery of measures. Trained study personnel also read the survey aloud to the participants in their classrooms. Compensation was not provided.

Measures

All measures were chosen based on prior use with children of similar ages. Details regarding each measure are provided below.

Parental psychological control

Parental psychological control was assessed using the 10-item Psychological Control Scale (Barber, 1996). This measure asks participants to report on the parent they spend the most time with and includes items such as "my parent is a person who changes the subject whenever I have something to say," and "my parent is a person who finishes my sentences whenever I talk." Responses ranged from 1 (Not Like My Parent) to 3 (A Lot Like My Parent). For the current study, mean scores were calculated with higher scores indicating greater perceived parental psychological control. The Psychological Control Scale is one of the most widely used measure of psychological control among children and adolescents (Barber et al., 2012). The measure has demonstrated concurrent and predictive validity for a range of youth mental health outcomes including depression and delinquency (Barber, 1996; Frazer & Fite, 2016). Previous studies that have used this measure with elementary school-aged children and adolescents and have found good validity (e.g., Blossom et al., 2016) and internal consistency (Fite et al., 2021). In the current sample the internal consistency for this measure was good (α = .87).

Functions of aggression

Proactive aggression and reactive aggression were assessed using Dodge and Coie (1987) 6-item Proactive and Reactive Scale. This measure has three items to assess proactive aggression (e.g., "I get other kids to gang up on somebody they do not like") and three items to assess reactive aggression (e.g., "I get angry easily when teased or threatened"). Responses ranged from 0 (Never) to 4 (Almost Always). Previous studies have used a two-factor measurement structure (i.e., proactive aggression, reactive aggression) and have found good validity (e.g., Dodge & Coie, 1987; Hubbard et al., 2010). This measure also has good internal consistency and high construct, concurrent, and content validity in children (Dodge & Coie, 1987; Fite et al., 2017) and has been used as a child self-report of aggression in both outpatient (Evans et al., 2019; Fite et al., 2017) and inpatient (Fite et al., 2009) settings. In the current sample, the internal consistency for this measure was adequate for proactive aggression (α = .77) and modest for reactive aggression (α = .68).

Anxiety symptoms

Participants self-reported their experiences of worried, scared, and nervous feelings using the Pediatric Anxiety Scale of the Patient-Reported Outcomes Measurement Information System (PROMIS Pediatric Short Form v.1.1 – Anxiety 8b; Irwin et al., 2010). This 8-item measure assesses youth's anxiety symptoms (e.g., "I felt like something awful might happen") on a 5-point Likert scale from 0 (Never) to 4 (Always). Mean scores were calculated with higher scores indicating higher levels of anxiety symptoms. Based on self-reported item banks developed by the National Institutes of Health, this measure is a brief and valid measure of youth anxiety (Irwin et al., 2010) and has been used previously among elementary- and middle-school aged youth (Diaz & Fite, 2019; Irwin et al., 2010). Irwin et al. (2010) found this measure to demonstrate good internal validity among youth ages 8 to 17 years, and internal consistency in the current study was good (α = .94).

Data analysis plan

SPSS statistical software (IBM, 2019) was utilized to conduct all analyses, and all variables were standardized prior to analyses to reduce multicollinearity and aid in interpretation of interaction effects. First, bivariate associations among study variables were examined via correlation analyses. Multiple regression analyses were then conducted to determine unique and interactive associations. A model in which reactive aggression was regressed on gender, age, and proactive aggression was first estimated. Anxiety symptoms and the interactive effects between parental psychological control and anxiety symptoms were then added as independent variables to the model. This same series of models were then estimated for proactive aggression. Note that statistically significant interactions were probed at high (+1 SD) and low (-1SD) levels of the moderator to determine the nature of the effects (Aiken & West, 1991).

Results

Descriptive statistics

Table 1 includes correlations and descriptive statistics (including means, standard deviations, minimum and maximum values) of study variables. Parental psychological control was positively correlated with anxiety symptoms, reactive aggression, and proactive aggression ($rs = .15 - .46$, $ps < .05$), such that high levels of psychological control were associated with high levels of anxiety symptoms and high levels of both aggression subtypes. Anxiety symptoms were positively linked to reactive ($r = .23$, $p < .05$), but not proactive, aggression, such that high levels of anxiety symptoms were associated with high levels of reactive aggression. Additionally, reactive and proactive aggression were moderately positively associated ($r = .37$, $p < .05$), suggesting that high levels of proactive aggression are associated with high levels of reactive aggression.

Multiple regression analyses

As reported in Table 2, when reactive aggression was regressed on proactive aggression, gender, age, and psychological control, gender was negatively ($\beta = -.15$, $p = .01$) and proactive aggression was positively ($\beta = .28$, $p = .00$) associated with reactive aggression. These findings indicated that boys reported higher levels of reactive aggression than girls and that high levels of proactive aggression were linked to high levels of reactive aggression. Further, parental psychological control was positively associated with reactive aggression ($\beta = .13$, $p = .02$), indicating that high levels of psychological control are linked to high levels of reactive aggression. Anxiety symptoms and the interaction between parental psychological control and anxiety symptoms were then added to the model. Anxiety symptoms were positively associated with reactive

Table 1. Correlations and descriptive statistics of study variables.

	1	2	3	4	5	6
1. Gender	–					
2. Age	−.03	–				
3. Psych. Control	.02	−.02	–			
4. Anxiety Symptoms	.21**	−.05	.46**	–		
5. Reactive Agg.	−.20**	−.10	.17**	.23**	–	
6. Proactive Agg.	−.15*	−.08	.15*	.02	.37**	–
Mean	–	12.30	1.33	.77	.77	.13
Standard Deviation	–	.92	.41	.91	.78	.46
Minimum	–	11.00	1.00	.00	.00	.00
Maximum	–	14.00	3.00	4.00	3.33	3.50

Note. Gender (1= Males, 2= Females). Psych. Control = Parental Psychological Control. Reactive Agg. = Reactive Aggression. Proactive Agg. = Proactive Aggression.
*$p < .05$.
**$p < .01$.

Table 2. Regression analyses.

	Reactive Aggression Models				Proactive Aggression Models			
	Without Anxiety and Interaction		With Anxiety and Interaction		Without Anxiety and Interaction		With Anxiety and Interaction	
	β	SE	β	SE	β	SE	β	SE
Gender	−.15**	.06	−.20**	.06	−.09	.06	−.06	.06
Age	−.08	.06	−.08	.05	−.05	.06	−.04	.06
Parental Psychological Control	.13*	.06	.03	.07	.10†	.06	.18**	.07
Other Function of Aggression	.28**	.06	.29**	.06	.29**	.06	.31**	.06
Anxiety Symptoms	–	–	.26**	.07	–	–	−.11	.07
Psychological Control X Anxiety	–	–	−.01	.05	–	–	−.06	.05

Note. Gender (0 = Males, 1= Females).
†$p < .08$.
*$p < .05$.
**$p < .01$.

aggression (β = .26, p = .00), but no interaction effects were evident (β = −.01, p = .84). These results suggest that while high levels of both anxiety symptoms and psychological control are linked to high levels of reactive aggression, their effects are unique and independent of one another.

Table 2 also includes analyses related to proactive aggression. Reactive aggression was positively associated with proactive aggression (β = .29, p = .00). Further, there was a marginally statistically significant trend indicating that parental psychological control was positively associated with proactive aggression (β = .10, p = .076), suggesting that high levels of psychological control are modestly linked to high levels of proactive aggression. Anxiety symptoms and the interaction between parental psychological control and anxiety symptoms were then added to the model, but no effects were evident (βs = −.11 & −.06, ps > .10). Findings suggest that the effects of psychological control on proactive aggression are not impacted by levels of anxiety symptoms.

Discussion

The present study advances the aggression literature by examining the links between parental psychological control and proactive and reactive functions of aggression in early adolescence. Findings suggested that parental psychological control was linked to both functions of aggression, but the link with reactive aggression was more robust than the link with proactive aggression. Further, anxiety symptoms were linked with reactive, not proactive, aggression, but anxiety symptoms did not impact the links between parental psychological control and the functions of aggression.

As noted above, parental psychological control was associated with both reactive and proactive aggression at the bivariate level. Further, when examining unique relations, psychological control was positively linked to reactive aggression and marginally statistically significantly positively related to proactive aggression. It appears that psychological control is more strongly linked to reactive aggression than proactive aggression. These findings are somewhat consistent with prior research that found that parental psychological control was only associated with youth self-reports of reactive, but not proactive, aggression (McClain et al., 2020). Parental psychological control may not provide a stable and consistent environment for youth to learn appropriate social cues and likely elicits poor emotional responding (Barber, 1996; Barber & Harmon, 2002), resulting in most commonly reactive aggression (McClain et al., 2020). Parental psychological control may also model ways of manipulating others (Barber, 1996; Barber & Harmon, 2002), which may result in both functions of aggression. However, further research is needed to further elucidate and confirm these findings before firm conclusions are drawn.

Also consistent with prior research (Barber & Harmon, 2002; Nanda et al., 2012), parental psychological control was positively associated with anxiety symptoms. Emotionally manipulating parenting associated with parental psychological control likely results in negative emotionality, including symptoms of anxiety.

Anxiety symptoms were uniquely associated with reactive aggression as expected and consistent with prior research (Card & Little, 2006; Vitaro et al., 2002). Anxiety symptoms and reactive aggression share similar physiological and social correlates and likely contribute to one another (Fite et al., 2016). Contrary to expectation and prior research (Wagner & Abaied, 2016), however, anxiety symptoms did not impact the influence of parental psychological control on either function of aggression. This contradictory finding may be due to different measures used, as the current study examined self-reported symptoms of anxiety compared to skin conductance responsivity. Further, this difference in the results could be due to the developmental period examined, as the current study focused on early adolescence and the prior study focused on emerging adults. Perhaps the impact of anxiety symptoms on these associations increase as youth age through adolescence. Finally, the prior study focused specifically on relational proactive and reactive aggression while the current measure of aggression assesses mostly physical aggression. It may be that the impact of anxiety in these associations is specific to relational forms of these functions of aggression. More research evaluating the role of anxiety symptoms is warranted before firm conclusions are drawn.

Implications, limitations, and future directions

The current study's findings should be interpreted while considering its limitations. First, this cross-sectional study limits the ability to draw causal conclusion regarding associations among parental psychological control and the functions of aggression. Future studies examining the longitudinal associations between psychological control and the functions of aggression across development would be useful to also contribute to our understanding of developmental timing of these associations. Further, this study relied solely on self-reported data. Future studies may benefit from having multiple informants, such as teacher-report, when assessing youth's proactive and reactive aggression. The current sample also reported relatively low rates of proactive aggression, reactive aggression, and anxiety symptoms. Future studies may consider examining these links among youth with elevated symptoms to speak to the generalizability of findings.

Nonetheless, the current study provides further evidence that that parental psychological control is maladaptive and contributes to both proactive and reactive functions of aggression, with a particularly strong link to reactive aggression, in addition to internalizing symptoms (i.e., anxiety symptoms). Further, these effects are evident during emerging adolescence, a time in which youth are experiencing increase social and emotional challenges (Hankin et al., 2010; Rudolph & Hammen, 1999). This pattern of findings may suggest that working on effective parenting strategies (including effective communication) during this age group can be particularly important in the prevention of aggressive behavior.

Disclosure statement

The authors report no conflicts of interest. The authors alone are responsible for the content and writing of the paper.

Ethical standards and informed consent

All procedures followed were in accordance with the ethical standards of the responsible committee on human experimentation [institutional and national] and with the Helsinki Declaration of 1975, as revised in 2000. Informed consent was obtained from all patients for being included in the study.

References

Aiken, L. S., & West, S. G. (1991). *Multiple regression: Testing and interpreting interactions*. Sage.

Bandura, A. (1973). *Aggression: A social learning analysis*. Prentice-Hall.

Barber, B. K. (1996). Parental psychological control: Revisiting a neglected construct. *Child Development, 67*(6), 3296–3319. https://doi.org/10.2307/1131780

Barber, B. K., & Harmon, E. L. (2002). Violating the self: Parental psychological control of children and adolescents. In B. K. Barber (Ed.), *Intrusive parenting: How psychological control affects children and adolescents* (pp. 15–52). APA.

Barber, B. K., Xia, M., Olsen, J. A., McNeely, C. A., & Bose, K. (2012). Feeling disrespected by parents: Refining the measurement and understanding of psychological control. *Journal of Adolescence, 35*(2), 273–287. https://doi.org/10.1016/j.adolescence.2011.10.010

Berkowitz, L. (1993). *Aggression: Its causes, consequences, and control*. Mcgraw-Hill Book Company.

Blossom, J. B., Fite, P. J., Frazer, A. L., Cooley, J. L., & Evans, S. C. (2016). Parental psychological control and aggression in youth: Moderating effect of emotion dysregulation. *Journal of Applied Developmental Psychology, 44*, 12–20. https://doi.org/10.1016/j.appdev.2016.02.006

Bronfenbrenner, U. (1977). Toward an experimental ecology of human development. *American Psychologist, 32*(7), 513–531. https://doi.org/10.1037/0003-066X.32.7.513

Card, N. A., & Little, T. D. (2006). Proactive and reactive aggression in childhood and adolescence: A meta-analysis of differential relations with psychosocial adjustment. *International Journal of Behavioral Development, 30*(5), 466–480. https://doi.org/10.1177/0165025406071904

Diaz, K., & Fite, P. (2019). Cyber victimization and its association with substance use, anxiety and depression symptoms among middle school youth. *Child and Youth Care Forum, 47*, 529–544. https://doi.org/10.1037/0022-3514.53.6.1146

Dodge, K. A., & Coie, J. D. (1987). Social-information-processing factors in reactive and proactive aggression in children's peer groups. *Journal of Personality and Social Psychology, 53*(6), 1146–1158. https://doi.org/10.1037/0022-3514.53.6.1146

Evans, S. C., Frazer, A. L., Blossom, J. B., & Fite, P. J. (2019). Forms and functions of aggression in early childhood. *Journal of Clinical Child & Adolescent Psychology, 48*, 790–798.

Fite, P. J., Stoppelbein, L., & Greening, L. (2009). Proactive and reactive aggression in a child psychiatric inpatient population. *Journal of Clinical Child & Adolescent Psychology, 38*(2), 199–205. https://doi.org/10.1080/15374410802698461

Fite, P. J., Craig, J., Colder, C. R., Lochman, J. E., & Wells, K. C. (2016). Proactive and reactive aggression. In R. J. R. Levesque (Ed.), *Encyclopedia of adolescence*. Springer International Publishing Switzerland.

Fite, P. J., Diaz, K. I., & Doyle, R. L. (2020). Does behavioral dysregulation moderate the links between contextual factors and substance use among detained youth? Advance online publication. *Journal of Child & Adolescent Substance Abuse, 29*, 143–154. https://doi.org/10.1080/1067828X.2021.1907265

Fite, P. J., Poquiz, J., Frazer, A. L., & Reiter, N. (2017). Further evaluation of associations between reactive and proactive aggression and suicidal behavior in a treatment seeking sample of youth. *Child Psychiatry & Human Development, 48*(6), 903–910. https://doi.org/10.1007/s10578-017-0713-4

Folkman, S., & Lazarus, R. S. (1984). *Stress, appraisal, and coping* (p. 460). Springer Publishing Company.

Frazer, A. L., & Fite, P. J. (2016). Maternal psychological control, use of supportive parenting, and childhood depressive symptoms. *Child Psychiatry and Human Development, 47*(3), 384–396. https://doi.org/10.1007/s10578-015-0573-8

Granic, I. (2014). The role of anxiety in the development, maintenance, and treatment of childhood aggression. *Development and Psychopathology, 26*(4 Pt 2), 1515–1530. https://doi.org/10.1017/S0954579414001175

Hankin, B. L., Stone, L., & Wright, P. A. (2010). Co-rumination, interpersonal stress generation, and internalizing symptoms: Accumulating effects and transactional influences in a multiwave study of adolescents. *Development and Psychopathology, 22*(1), 217–235. https://doi.org/10.1017/S0954579409990368

Hubbard, J. A., McAuliffe, M. D., Morrow, M. T., & Romano, L. J. (2010). Reactive and proactive aggression in childhood and adolescence: Precursors, outcomes, processes, experiences, and measurement. *Journal of Personality, 78*(1), 95–118. https://doi.org/10.1111/j.1467-6494.2009.00610.x

IBM. (2019). *IBM SPSS statistics for windows, Version 26.0.* IBM Corp.

Irwin, D. E., Stucky, B., Langer, M. M., Thissen, D., DeWitt, E. M., Lai, J. S., Varni, J. W., Yeatts, K., & DeWalt, D. A. (2010). An item response analysis of the pediatric PROMIS anxiety and depressive symptoms scales. *Quality of Life Research: An International Journal of Quality of Life Aspects of Treatment, Care and Rehabilitation, 19*(4), 595–607. https://doi.org/10.1007/s11136-010-9619-3

Kuppens, S., Laurent, L., Heyvaert, M., & Onghena, P. (2013). Associations between parental psychological control and relational aggression in children and adolescents: A multilevel and sequential meta-analysis. *Developmental Psychology, 49*(9), 1697–1712. https://doi.org/10.1037/a0030740

Lamarche, V., Brendgen, M., Boivin, M., Vitaro, F., Dionne, G., & Pérusse, D. (2007). Do friends' characteristics moderate the prospective links between peer victimization and reactive and proactive aggression? *Journal of Abnormal Child Psychology, 35*(4), 665–680. https://doi.org/10.1007/s10802-007-9122-7

Loukas, A., Paulos, S. K., & Robinson, S. (2005). Early adolescent social and overt aggression: Examining the roles of social anxiety and maternal psychological control. *Journal of Youth and Adolescence, 34*(4), 335–345. https://doi.org/10.1007/s10964-005-5757-2

McClain, C. M., Manring, S., Frazer, A. L., Elledge, L. C., & Fite, P. J. (2020). The moderating effects of child-perceived parental psychological control on the association between functions of aggression and peer victimization in elementary school children. *Journal of Psychopathology and Behavioral Assessment, 42*, 281–295. https://doi.org/10.1007/s10862-019-09771-w

Nanda, M. M., Kotchick, B. A., & Grover, R. L. (2012). Parental psychological control and childhood anxiety: The mediating role of perceived lack of control. *Journal of Child and Family Studies, 21*(4), 637–645. https://doi.org/10.1007/s10826-011-9516-6

Pinquart, M. (2017a). Associations of parenting dimensions and styles with externalizing problems of children and adolescents: An updated meta-analysis. *Developmental Psychology, 53*(5), 873–932. http://dx.doi.org/10.1037/dev0000295

Pinquart, M. (2017b). Associations of parenting dimensions and styles with internalizing symptoms in children and adolescents: A meta-analysis. *Marriage & Family Review, 53*(7), 613–640. https://doi.org/10.1080/01494929.2016.1247761

Rathert, J., Fite, P. J., Gaertner, A. E., & Vitulano, M. (2011). Associations between effortful control, psychological control and proactive and reactive aggression. *Child Psychiatry and Human Development, 42*(5), 609–621. https://doi.org/10.1007/s10578-011-0236-3

Rudolph, K. D., & Hammen, C. (1999). Age and gender as determinants of stress exposure, generation, and reactions in youngsters: A transactional perspective. *Child Development, 70*(3), 660–677. https://doi.org/10.1111/1467-8624.00048

Vitaro, F., Barker, E. D., Boivin, M., Brendgen, M., & Tremblay, R. E. (2006). Do early difficult temperament and harsh parenting differentially predict reactive and proactive aggression? *Journal of Abnormal Child Psychology, 34*(5), 681–691. https://doi.org/10.1007/s10802-006-9055-6

Vitaro, F., Brendgen, M., & Tremblay, R. E. (2002). Reactively and proactively aggressive children: Antecedent and subsequent characteristics. *Journal of Child Psychology and Psychiatry, and Allied Disciplines, 43*(4), 495–505. https://doi.org/10.1111/1469-7610.00040

Wagner, C. R., & Abaied, J. L. (2016). Skin conductance level reactivity moderates the association between parental psychological control and relational aggression in emerging adulthood. *Journal of Youth and Adolescence, 45*(4), 687–700. https://doi.org/10.1007/s10964-016-0422-5

Perpetration of intimate partner violence and guilt: The role of parenting status

Emily C. Taverna, Devin J. McGuier and Amy D. Marshall

ABSTRACT

A paucity of research addresses individual differences in the experience of moral emotions (e.g., guilt) related to one's intimate partner violence (IPV) perpetration. Because IPV exposure negatively impacts children, we examined whether IPV perpetration is differentially associated with guilt for parents and non-parents. We conducted multilevel regression analyses among 103 individuals from 52 heterosexual community couples. Parent status moderated the association, such that *non-parents* reported greater overall, state, and trait guilt in association with greater IPV perpetration whereas parents did not. Parent status did not moderate the relations between IPV victimization and guilt, suggesting that this result is specific to perpetration. We further observed differences with regard to emotion regulation, such that parents had greater difficulty attending to their emotions. Parents may exhibit muted guilt in relation to their perpetration, potentially due to difficulty attending to their emotions. Because guilt in relation to IPV perpetration is a relatively new area of study, research is needed to further elucidate the mechanisms and directionality of this relationship. Current findings suggest that emotion regulation strategies that foster healthy processing of guilt may be important considerations for IPV prevention and intervention research, particularly those that address vulnerability for IPV during the transition to parenthood.

Intimate partner violence (IPV) is highly prevalent in the United States (McKinney et al., 2009) and is associated with a range of mental health problems for victims (E. Lawrence et al., 2012) and child witnesses (e.g., Artz et al., 2014). Studies have consistently documented links between IPV victimization and mental health disorders (Spencer et al., 2019) as well as intense emotions such as guilt (Ansara & Hindin, 2011). Less work has focused on delineating mental health and emotional correlates of IPV perpetration. What work does exist in this area has typically considered emotional experiences such as shame (A. Lawrence & Taft, 2013) to be predictors, rather than consequences, of IPV perpetration. However, IPV is commonly a dyadic phenomenon such that bidirectional IPV is the most prevalent pattern (49–70%; Langhinrichsen-Rohling et al., 2012) and negative behaviors reciprocally escalate between partners (Burman et al., 1993). Thus, there exists a need to tease apart the degree to which emotional experiences are associated with IPV perpetration compared to IPV victimization. In particular, associations with IPV perpetration must be examined when considering emotional experiences that may facilitate behavioral change, such as guilt.

Guilt refers to a distressing emotional response to self-reflection of one's transgressions or failures (e.g., Jones et al., 2000). Although excessive or otherwise inappropriate feelings of guilt are problematic and symptomatic of a number of disorders (most notably major depressive disorder; American Psychiatric Association, 2013), appropriate experiences of guilt are crucial for promoting behavioral change and adaptive styles of conflict resolution following perceived transgressions (Baumeister et al., 1995; Tangney et al., 2011; Tracy & Robins, 2006). While the effect of IPV perpetration on feelings of guilt has yet to be studied, when other forms of violence perpetration (e.g., violence perpetration in the context of military service) have been examined, moral emotions (including guilt) have been identified as common consequences of violence perpetration (e.g., Dennis et al., 2017).

In addition to better understanding associations between IPV perpetration and guilt, there is a need to understand how individual differences, such as parent status, impact these associations. The transition to parenthood is marked by increased stress, marital dissatisfaction, and conflict (Doss et al., 2009; E. Lawrence et al., 2008). With this, rates of IPV peak during the early years of parenting (Gustafsson & Cox, 2016) and children may be victimized during incidents of IPV (e.g., Mbilinyi et al., 2007). Children exposed to IPV often experience a range of negative outcomes, including mental and physical health problems, cognitive impairments, and academic difficulties (Artz et al., 2014).

To our knowledge, no studies have examined whether parents and non-parents differentially experience guilt or other moral emotions following IPV perpetration. However, complex relational dynamics associated with parenthood suggests that parents may experience IPV differently than non-parents. The transition to parenthood involves a transition from a dyadic system (partner to partner) to an increasingly complex family system composed of multiple relationships including partner to partner, parent to child, and partner to child. Stress and trauma experienced between two members of the family system (e.g., IPV) can reverberate to impact relationships between other members of the family system (Feinberg, 2003; Minuchin, 1985). Thus, consequences of IPV may be more widespread for parents than for non-parents due to the impact on multiple members of the family system, potentially increasing feelings of guilt.

In addition to inhabiting more complex family systems, parents may face greater regulatory demands compared to non-parents, which may limit their ability to regulate distressing emotions, including guilt. Parents must regulate their own emotions (and to an extent their partner's emotions) while also supporting their children's emotional development (Eisenberg et al., 1998; Hajal & Paley, 2020). Parenthood may also "raise the stakes" of emotion regulation, as parents are often required to regulate their own emotions (particularly distressing emotions) in order to maintain positive, responsive interactions with their children (e.g., Rutherford et al., 2015). While this is crucial for supporting children's development, parents' emotion regulation capacities may become overburdened under significant stress, resulting in failure to adequately regulate their own and their children's emotions (Crandall et al., 2015).

These emotion regulation differences may limit parents' ability to cope effectively with stress. A variety of factors may contribute to stress and reduced well-being among parents, such as social support and financial resources (e.g., Raikes & Thompson, 2005). Some stress theories suggest that stressors are situations that are perceived to threaten individuals' resources of instrumental or personal value, and that accumulation of stressors may increase the likelihood of resources being depleted (Hobfoll, 2001). In application of this theory, the range of potential consequences related to IPV may contribute to an accumulation of stress (i.e., conflict-related stress and parenting stress) and greater deterioration of resources (i.e., regulating own emotions and child's emotions). Taken together, the increased regulatory demands faced by parents, particularly during periods of high stress, may limit their ability to regulate their own distressing emotions (including guilt following perpetration of IPV).

Despite the potential for parent status to impact feelings of guilt following IPV perpetration, little research exists in this area. Studies have generally failed to examine parents' experience of guilt following IPV. However, witnessing IPV is linked to a host of problematic outcomes for children, and a small body of literature indicates that parents who perpetrate and/or experience IPV are aware of the negative consequences of witnessing IPV for their children (Rhodes et al., 2010; Rothman et al., 2007; see Salisbury et al., 2009 for contradictory findings). Furthermore, parents have been shown to experience guilt related to children's mental health problems generally (McDonald et al., 2007; Richert et al., 2018). These findings may suggest that parents' knowledge that IPV can negatively impact their children may result in parents experiencing greater guilt following perpetration of IPV than non-parents.

We examined potential differences between parents and non-parents in the relations between IPV perpetration and guilt. Given that interventions for IPV perpetration are generally ineffective (Eckhardt et al., 2013), this area of research may inform a potential mechanism of change that could be addressed within parenting interventions for IPV. Consistent with aforementioned research documenting that experiencing guilt is crucial for promoting behavioral change (Baumeister et al., 1995; Tangney et al., 2011; Tracy & Robins, 2006), understanding whether parents have unique experiences of guilt may inform how to best address this emotion based on family structure (e.g., couples with and without children). Other areas of research examining stress among parents specifically suggest that parental guilt may mitigate the impact of parental stressors (e.g., work interference with family, needs frustration) on parenting behavior (Cho & Allen, 2012; Slobodin et al., 2020), suggesting that this may be a similarly useful emotion to examine in the context of IPV to reduce the impact of this behavior on victims and child witnesses.

In framing our hypotheses, we operated from a cognitive-behavioral theoretical perspective, such that we view discrete emotional states, such as guilt, to increase or decrease the use of behaviors via intrinsically reinforcing or punishing effects. We hypothesized that parent status would moderate a positive association between degree of IPV perpetration and severity of experienced guilt. We formed this hypothesis on the basis that parents may feel broader effects of their behavior not only for themselves and their partners, but also for their children, and that the stress and increased regulatory demands placed on parents may reduce their ability to regulate their own distressing emotions (including guilt). Although IPV perpetration was our primary focus, we examined separate models of IPV perpetration and victimization. As IPV victimization and perpetration often co-occur, we aimed to demonstrate that the relationship with guilt is specific to perpetration and not due to the co-occurrence of victimization, which would lend support to the proposed hypothesis. In addition to the overall experience of guilt, we examined subscales capturing recent guilt, persistent guilt, and moral standards, to help infer the temporal relationship of guilt and IPV perpetration. We also conducted post-hoc analyses to explore differences between parents and nonparents in terms of emotion regulation abilities to help interpret our observations.

Method

Participants and procedures

Participants included heterosexual couples who were recruited from rural or semi-rural Pennsylvania communities between 2008 and 2010 via advertisements within the local community (e.g., flyers in mental health clinics, newspaper advertisements). Interested participants completed a phone screen to confirm eligibility. To be included in the study, partners needed to be cohabitating and over the age of 18. The data were initially collected to examine associations between trauma and relationship conflict, and at least one partner in each couple had to meet screening criteria for post-traumatic stress disorder (PTSD) using the Posttraumatic Checklist (Weathers et al., 1993). PTSD symptom severity was assessed for all participants via the Clinician Administered PTSD Scale (CAPS; Blake et al., 1995) during the study session. In total, 64 couples (128 individuals) were eligible and completed the study procedures. Following approval by the Institutional Review Board at The Pennsylvania State University (study #27507), all participants provided written informed consent in person at the beginning of their first laboratory session. Participants completed either one eight hour or two four-hour lab sessions, as well as take home questionnaires. The current study analyses were limited to participants with complete data on measures utilized in this study ($n = 103$; 48 men, 55 women).

Couples with a combined annual income greater than $100,000 or a partner with six or more years of post-high school education were excluded from this sample to avoid inclusion of university faculty and others who may not be representative of the larger community. Each participant completed a measure of demographics and a measure of IPV victimization and perpetration during an in-person lab session. Measures of experienced guilt and difficulties with emotion regulation were completed at home, then returned at the second laboratory session or via mail. Participants provided informed consent and received $175 for completion of the full protocol, including procedures not included herein.

The majority of participants identified as White or Caucasian (85.4%), and 6.8% identified as African American, 3.9% as Hispanic/Latino, and 3.9% as bi-racial/multi-racial. Participants had a mean age of 37.72 years ($SD = 13.02$), monthly income of $1,660.72 ($SD$ = $1,482.20), and education level of 14.22 years ($SD = 2.27$), with the majority of participants being employed (71.3%). Most couples were married (71%) and average relationship length was 12 years and 9 months ($SD = 11$ years, 11 months). Most participants (65%) were parents.

Measures

Parent status

Participants reported the 1) number of children they have had or adopted with their current partner, 2) number of children from other relationships, and 3) number of other children living in their home. A dichotomous parent status variable was created, such that those who indicated being responsible for *any* children were considered to be a parent, and all others were considered non-parents. Complete information about the child(ren)'s residential status was not available, so it is possible that not all parents had children living in the home.

Intimate partner violence

Physical intimate partner violence experienced and perpetrated during the past year was assessed using the 12-item physical aggression subscale from the Revised Conflict Tactics Scales (CTS2; Straus et al., 1996), which demonstrates internal consistency and test-retest reliability (Straus et al., 1996; Vega & O'Leary, 2007) and convergent and discriminant validity (Slep & O'Leary, 2005; Straus et al., 1996). Participants rated how often they and their partner engaged in each act of aggression (e.g., kicking, beating up) within the past year. Per recommendations by Moffitt and colleagues (1997), we used a "variety score" that indicates how many different acts of physical aggression (of the 12 assessed) occurred. This scoring method is favored because it reduces potential problems with the reliability of the response format as a consequence of number of occurrences over the past year being more difficult for participants to report than whether the act occurred (Moffitt et al., 1997). In addition, this variable is theoretically consistent with the proposed models. That is, individuals who engaged in a greater variety of behaviors may more readily recognize that they engage in problematic conflict behaviors that induce guilt, as opposed to individuals who engage in many instances of one type of behavior, which they may not recognize as problematic. We also selected physical aggression rather than other forms of aggression because these behaviors are often more severe and participants were thought to more readily recognize these behaviors as wrong, whereas attributions for psychological aggression may be more variable and ambiguous for many individuals. For cases in which partners disagreed about whether a violent behavior was perpetrated, we applied either the individual's self-report of their own perpetration or the partner's report of their own victimization, depending on which partner endorsed the behavior occurring (Slep & O'Leary, 2005). Internal consistency was adequate for the perpetration ($\alpha = 0.43$ men; $\alpha = 0.70$ women) and victimization (α = .72 for men; α = .66 for women) subscales.

Guilt

The Guilt Inventory (Jones et al., 2000) consists of three subscales, with items rated on a 5-point Likert scale ranging from 1 (*Strongly Agree*) to 5 (*Strongly Disagree*). The 10-item State Guilt scale assesses experiences of guilt due to recent behavior (e.g., "I have recently done something that

I deeply regret"). The 20-item Trait Guilt subscale assesses experiences of guilt related to past events (e.g., "There is something in my past that I deeply regret"). The 15-item Moral Standards subscale assesses moral beliefs (e.g., "I feel a strong need to live up to my moral values"). Due to the nature of the measure, a time frame for recent or past behaviors was not specified; rather, these attributions were made by the participant when responding. The measure also captures general experiences of guilt and is not anchored specifically to IPV perpetration. Internal consistency was good for the overall measure (α = .90 for men; α = .85 for women), as well as the state (α = .78 for men; α = .74 for women), trait (α = .91 for men; α = .87 for women), and moral (α = .66 for men; α = .78 for women) subscales.

Emotion regulation

The 36-item Difficulties in Emotion Regulation Scale (DERS; Gratz & Roemer, 2004) is comprised of six subscales pertaining to emotion dysregulation: 1) nonacceptance of one's distress, 2) difficulties engaging in goal-directed behavior, 3) impulse control difficulties when experiencing distress, 4) lack of emotional awareness, 5) limited emotion regulation strategies, and 6) lack of emotional clarity about the emotions one is experiencing. Responses are rated from 1 (*Almost Never*) to 5 (*Almost Always*), and all subscales are scored such that higher scores indicate greater emotion regulation difficulty. The measure is both reliable and valid (e.g., Gratz & Roemer, 2004), and Cronbach's alpha in the current study was .93 for both men and women (subscales ranged from .79 to .91 for men and from .81 to .92 for women). Three subscales each contained one outlier based on the means and standard deviations within groups (i.e., parents and non-parents). These individuals were excluded from analyses pertaining to emotion regulation difficulties.

Demographics

Participants self-reported their age in years and gender during the study session. Age was grand-mean centered and gender was effect coded (men = −1 and women = 1).

Statistical analyses

The Guilt Inventory was completed by participants at home and, consequently, was completed and returned by only 81% of participants ($n = 103$; 48 men, 55 women). One additional participant had more than 20% of items missing on each subscale and another participant had more than 20% of items missing for the moral guilt subscale, and were excluded from analyses involving the indicated scale. There were no statistically significant differences between those who completed the GI and those who did not with regard to parent status or other demographic variables (all p values > 0.213). Mean replacement was used when fewer than 20% of items were missing on a single scale. To examine the appropriateness of handling missing data in this manner, we also utilized multiple imputation to estimate missing data, then analyzed the resulting full dataset and report comparability of results across methods.

Because men and women are nested within couples, descriptive and correlational analyses were run separately for men and women to avoid potential problems related to dependency within couples. Next, multilevel regression analyses were conducted using the lme4 package available through R statistical software (Bates et al., 2014). Two-level models were specified with individuals nested in couples such that the couple level error term accounts for systematic variability stemming from partners being nested within couples. To examine the amount of variance attributed to the person and the amount of variance attributed to the couple, for each outcome (i.e., total guilt and each guilt subscale), a variance decomposition null model was calculated including no predictors at Level 1 (individuals) or Level 2 (couples). Another model was then created including the main effects of parent status, IPV perpetration or victimization, the interaction between parent status and IPV perpetration/victimization, and covariates (i.e., gender, age) included as additional Level 1 predictors. In all models, we controlled for the main effect of parent age because older parents are less likely to have children living in the home. To explore differences between parents and non-parents with regard to emotion regulation difficulties, we tested additional models including parenting status as a Level 1 predictor of overall difficulties in emotion regulation and each of the DERS subscales.

Results

Descriptive analyses

In the current sample, 62% of women and 69% of men reported being parents. Parents and non-parents significantly differed with regard to age, such that parents ($M = 41.46$ years, $SD = 11.47$) were older than non-parents ($M = 30.77$ years, $SD = 13.01$; $t = 2.51$, $p = .014$) but there was not a significant difference between parents ($M = 188.12$ months, $SD = 143.84$) and non-parents ($M = 86.79$ months, $SD = 119.01$) with regard to relationship length ($t = 1.06$, $p = .294$). At least one act of physical IPV was perpetrated by 29% of participants (36% of women; 21% of men) in the past year. Of the participants who met diagnostic criteria for PTSD via the CAPS ($N = 37$), similar numbers of parents ($N = 21$) and non-parents ($N = 16$) met diagnostic criteria; however, non-parents ($M = 42.78$, $SD = 25.14$) experienced marginally significantly greater symptom severity than parents ($M = 33.27$, $SD = 22.33$; $t = -1.97$, $p = 0.051$, $d = 0.42$). Furthermore, there were no statistically significant differences between parents and non-parents with respect to overall guilt ($t = -1.02$, $p = 0.309$, $d = 0.22$), state guilt ($t = -0.44$, $p = 0.749$, $d = 0.07$), trait guilt ($t = -1.69$, $p = 0.095$, $d = 0.36$) or moral guilt ($t = 0.65$, $p = 0.517$, $d = 0.09$).

Table 1 presents descriptive statistics and bivariate correlations among study variables. In the overall sample, the average number of physically aggressive acts perpetrated was 0.69 ($SD = 1.31$) out of twelve possible acts assessed ($M = 0.84$; $SD = 1.37$ among women; $M = 0.52$; $SD = 1.24$ among men). Among those who perpetrated IPV ($N = 30$), the average number of types of physically aggressive acts perpetrated was 2.37 ($SD = 1.40$). Among men who perpetrated IPV, the average number of types of physically aggressive acts was 2.50 ($SD = 1.58$) compared to 2.30 ($SD = 1.34$) among women who perpetrated IPV. There were no significant differences in men and women's IPV perpetration ($t = 1.91$, $p = .063$, $d = 0.18$), nor were there significant differences in parents' and non-parents' IPV perpetration ($t = -0.08$, $p = 0.195$, $d = .40$). The average overall guilt score in the current sample was 141.45 ($SD = 19.88$) out of a possible 225, with women ($M = 144.44$, $SD = 19.27$) experiencing similar levels of guilt as men ($M = 138.08$, $SD = 20.23$; $t = -1.63$, $p = .107$, $d = 0.32$). IPV perpetration and victimization were highly correlated for men ($r = 0.70$) and women ($r = 0.72$). IPV perpetration was not significantly correlated with overall guilt or any of the other guilt subscales among either men or women. State and trait guilt were highly correlated among men ($r = .79$) and women ($r = .74$). Moral guilt was not significantly correlated with either state or trait guilt.

Multilevel regression analyses

Examination of null models indicated that sufficient variance existed in each outcome to be predicted (all p values $< .001$) and that accounting for nesting within couples was necessary. First, we examined the impact of parent status, physical IPV perpetration, and their interaction on reported guilt (Table 2). Age and gender were included as covariates in all models though neither variable significantly predicted overall guilt or any of the guilt subscales. Similarly, the main effects of parent status and physical IPV perpetration did not significantly predict overall

Table 1. Descriptive statistics and intercorrelations among study variables.

Variable	1	2	3	4	5	6	*M*	*SD*	*n*	Range
1. IPV Perpetration	–	.72**	.10	.08	.05	.08	0.84	1.37	55	5.00
2. IPV Victimization	.70**	–	.22	.07	.17	.19	0.64	1.31	55	5.00
3. Overall guilt	.17	.13	–	.79**	.88**	.34*	144.44	19.27	54	86.73
4. State guilt	.11	.16	.85**	–	.74**	–.10	29.26	6.48	54	29.00
5. Trait guilt	.09	.07	.94**	.79**	–	–.09	63.72	12.73	54	52.00
6. Moral guilt	.25	.11	.41**	.06	.14	–	51.53	8.41	53	37.07
M	0.52	.75	138.08	27.67	60.34	50.09	–			
SD	1.24	1.36	20.23	6.63	12.86	6.13		–		
n	48	48	48	48	48	48			–	
Range	6.00	6.00	75.00	24.00	51.00	28.00				–

Notes. Women's correlations and descriptive statistics are presented above the diagonal; men's correlations and descriptive statistics are presented below the diagonal. Maximum possible scores were 225 for overall guilt, 50 for state guilt, 100 for trait guilt, and 75 for moral guilt. For each of these scales, higher numbers reflect greater guilt.

*$p < .05$.

**$p < .01$.

***$p < .001$.

Table 2. Multilevel regression models of IPV and parent status on reported guilt.

		Perpetration			Victimization		
Outcome	Predictor	B	*SE*	*t*	B	*SE*	*t*
Overall Guilt	Intercept	139.74	2.36	59.10***	139.71	2.40	58.15***
	Parent status	−2.02	5.06	0.40	−0.47	5.12	−0.09
	IPV	2.41	1.61	1.50	2.53	1.58	1.60
	IPV x Parent status	−6.55	3.08	−2.12*	−3.13	3.01	−1.04
State Guilt	Intercept	27.85	0.77	36.13***	227.87	0.79	35.29***
	Parent status	2.81	1.65	1.70	2.09	1.68	1.25
	IPV	0.53	0.53	1.00	0.51	0.52	0.99
	IPV x Parent status	−2.82	1.01	−2.80**	−1.82	0.99	−1.84
Trait Guilt	Intercept	61.65	1.52	40.68***	61.47	1.54	39.90***
	Parent status	0.28	3.25	0.09	−1.06	3.28	−0.32
	IPV	0.71	1.03	0.69	1.03	1.01	1.01
	IPV x Parent status	−4.39	1.98	−2.22*	−2.63	1.92	−1.36
Moral Guilt	Intercept	50.22	1.00	50.12***	50.47	1.01	50.05***
	Parent status	−0.54	2.07	−0.26	−1.27	2.06	−0.61
	IPV	1.05	0.61	1.72	0.76	0.59	1.28
	IPV x Parent status	0.40	1.17	0.34	1.42	1.13	1.26

Notes. Participants' grand mean centered age and gender (men = -1, women = 1) are included as covariates in all models. Parent status is coded as non-parents = -0.5 and parents = 0.5. B = unstandardized coefficient. *SE* = standard error.
*$p < .05$.
**$p < .01$.
***$p < .001$.

guilt or any of the guilt subscales. However, the interaction between parent status and physical IPV perpetration significantly predicted overall guilt, state guilt, and trait guilt (see Table 2 and Figure 1). Simple slopes analyses indicated that non-parents who have perpetrated a greater variety of IPV behaviors reported significantly more overall guilt (B = 5.68, *SE* = 2.45, *t* = 2.32), such that for every one additional type of IPV behavior used, non-parents reported a nearly six unit increase in overall guilt. Similarly, non-parents also had greater state guilt in relation to a greater variety of IPV behaviors (B = 1.93, *SE* = 0.80, *t* = 2.42), suggesting that for every one additional IPV behavior type used, non-parents demonstrate a nearly two unit increase in state guilt. Finally, the results were again similar for trait guilt (B = 2.91, *SE* = 2.91, *t* = 1.85), such that for every one additional type of IPV behavior used, non-parents demonstrated a nearly three unit increase in trait guilt scores. Among parents, simple slope analyses revealed that overall guilt (B = −0.87, *SE* = 1.98, *t* = −0.44), state guilt (B = −0.88, *SE* = 0.65, *t* = −1.37), and trait guilt (B = −1.48, *SE* = 1.27, *t* = −1.17) were not significantly associated with the variety of IPV behaviors perpetrated. The two-way interaction was statistically non-significant when predicting moral guilt. The pattern of results remains the same, albeit slightly smaller effect sizes, when using multiple imputation to account for missing data. In addition, removing outliers on the IPV variable did not change the pattern of results, thus we retained them in analyses because this reflects meaningful variability in aggression.

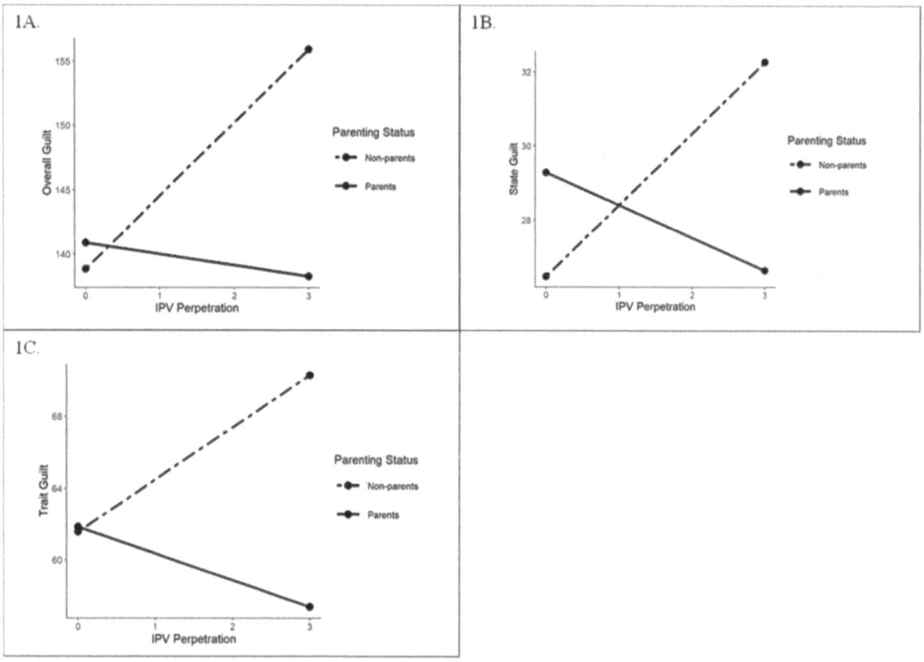

Figure 1. IPV perpetration significantly predicts total guilt (A), state guilt (B), and trait guilt (C) among non-parents, but not among parents.

Next, we examined parent status as a potential moderator of the effect of physical IPV victimization on reported guilt (Table 2). Age and gender were included as covariates in all models though neither variable predicted overall guilt or any of the guilt subscales. Similarly, the main effects and the interaction between parent status and physical IPV victimization were not significantly associated with overall guilt or any guilt subscales. The pattern of results remains the same when using multiple imputation to account for missing data.

Supplemental analyses

Multilevel regression analyses predicting the total DERS and each subscale by parent status (Table 3) suggested that non-parents ($M = 13.56$, SD = 4.56) had less difficulty attending to their emotions compared to parents ($M = 15.46$, SD = 4.52, $t = 2.03$). No other significant differences emerged. The pattern of results did not change when the models were examined using the original emotion regulation variables, when outliers were truncated to the next highest value, or when multiple imputation was used to account for missing data.

Table 3. Differences in emotion regulation difficulties and guilt between parents and non-parents.

	Parents		Non-parents				
	M	*SD*	*M*	*SD*	B	*SE*	*t*
DERS Scale							
Total Difficulties	76.99	21.48	79.21	21.13	−2.23	4.41	−0.50
Nonacceptance	11.76	4.83	12.17	4.39	−0.41	0.97	−0.42
Awareness	15.48	4.55	13.58	4.63	1.89	0.95	2.00*
Impulsivity	11.18	4.49	10.50	3.70	0.69	0. 90	0.77
Goal Directed Behavior	13.13	5.26	14.91	5.54	−1.78	1.11	−1.60
Strategies	15.17	6.13	16.79	6.74	−1.62	1.32	−1.23
Lack of emotional clarity	9.96	3.21	10.23	3.30	−0.27	0.68	−0.40
Guilt Inventory							
Overall Guilt	139.99	20.37	144.23	18.90	−4.24	4.15	−1.02
State Guilt	28.36	6.72	28.80	6.36	−0.44	1.38	−0.32
Trait Guilt	60.59	13.14	65.07	11.87	−4.48	2.65	−1.69
Moral Guilt	51.10	7.42	50.37	7.48	1.13	1.73	0.65

Notes. Parent status is coded as non-parents = −0.5 and parents = 0.5. B = unstandardized coefficient. *SE* = standard error.
*$p < .05$.
**$p < .01$.
***$p < .001$.

Discussion

The current study contributes to a limited literature documenting the relation between IPV perpetration and moral emotions, particularly as it differs between parents and non-parents. We hypothesized that guilt would be stronger among parents who perpetrate IPV than among non-parents, due to the potential for IPV to negatively impact the individual, their partner, *and* their children (e.g., Artz et al., 2014; E. Lawrence et al., 2012), parenting stress creating vulnerability to distressing emotions (e.g., Doss et al., 2009), and increased regulatory demands associated with parenting (Eisenberg et al., 1998; Hajal & Paley, 2020). This hypothesis was not supported. While substantial literature suggests that there is a positive association between IPV perpetration and constructs closely related to guilt (e.g., shame; A. Lawrence & Taft, 2013), results from this study suggest that the parenting role may limit awareness of feelings of guilt related to IPV perpetration. That is, in the current study, non-parents demonstrated a pattern consistent with this prior literature and appeared to have greater guilt with more IPV perpetrated. In contrast, parents did not appear to have elevated guilt in association with greater IPV perpetration. Although these results should be interpreted with caution and will warrant additional empirical investigation prior to drawing conclusions, we draw from prior research to identify possible theoretical explanations for these findings.

Although speculative, results suggest subtle differences in emotion regulation capacities between parents and non-parents that may contribute to parents' muted guilt responses following perpetration of IPV. We found that while parents and non-parents were similar in overall emotion regulation difficulties, parents reported poorer awareness of their emotions. This is consistent with prior research on parenting and emotion regulation (e.g., Rutherford et al., 2015). Indeed, it may be that parents fail to attend to their own distressing emotions because they are attending to their children's needs. This assertion is consistent with literature indicating that with parenthood, individuals' cognitive processes become preoccupied with thoughts about their child (Leckman et al., 2004). Meanwhile, non-parents may have more opportunity to attend to their own distressing emotions, potentially making their experience of guilt more salient.

Importantly, we did not find evidence that parents and non-parents differ with respect to other potential emotion regulation difficulties. Parents and non-parents did not demonstrate baseline differences with respect to many of the other observed variables (i.e., relationship length, PTSD severity, guilt subscales, extent of IPV perpetration). Although parents differed with respect to age, this was controlled for in the models. Taken together, this would suggest that parents and non-parents do not have substantial baseline differences in this sample that may be driving parents' muted guilt response.

One possible explanation for the muted guilt response in relation to IPV perpetration among parents is that parenting stress may tax a unique aspect of their emotion regulation capacity, that parents reported having greater difficulties with (i.e., emotional awareness). This is consistent with stress theories (Hobfoll, 2001), which posit that accumulation of stressors may deplete personal resources to cope with subsequent stressors. Parenthood is associated with a range of acute and chronic stressors (Deater-Deckard, 2008), and parenting stress may be heightened for those within conflictual intimate relationships (Owen et al., 2006). Thus, stress theories may help explain the observed results, such that both the stress of parenting and the experience of guilt may uniquely tax cognitive-emotional resources. To conserve resources, parents may be motivated to use avoidant coping in response their uncomfortable moral emotions, which could decrease awareness of guilt. Avoidant coping is thought to function to reduce distressing emotions related to violence perpetration, such as guilt, but may prevent appropriate resolution of the distress over time (Litz et al., 2009). Non-parents, on the other hand, may have greater capacity to tolerate distressing emotions because they have fewer additional demands (i.e., caring for children) straining their cognitive and emotional resources.

It is likely that the observed emotional correlates of IPV perpetration operate bi-directionally. That is, the positive associations consistently observed between emotion regulation difficulties and IPV perpetration (e.g., McNulty & Hellmuth, 2008) may indicate that aggression is a maladaptive strategy for regulating distressing emotions (Bushman et al., 2001). In turn, perpetration of IPV may heighten the presence of difficult moral emotions, as seen with other forms of violence perpetration (e.g., Dennis et al., 2017). Deficits in emotional awareness following perpetration may result in failure to attend to these moral emotions, as appears to be the case for parents. Understanding of these patterns could help elucidate why incidents of IPV often occur repeatedly among some couples (Testa et al., 2003). For example, avoidance of distressing emotions may not be sustainable over time, and in moments when chronic guilt is more salient, it may serve as an antecedent for aggressive behavior, whereas individuals who are able to tolerate their feelings of guilt may be less likely to repeat that behavior to prevent greater emotional distress. Understanding these patterns may also explain why the transition to parenthood confers increased risk for IPV (Gustafsson & Cox, 2016).

The current study is among the first to examine how parents and non-parents may differentially respond to their perpetration of aggression and proposes potential theories as to how this may inform IPV. It is our hope that this will serve as a preliminary investigation to inform emotional consequences of IPV and to differentiate processes among parents and non-parents. Although more research is needed to corroborate and expand these findings, results from this study suggest several important clinical implications. While experiences of guilt are distressing, they are also crucial mechanisms for promoting behavioral change and have been linked to adaptive patterns of conflict resolution, including apologies and attempts to make amends (Baumeister et al., 1995; Tangney et al., 2011; Tracy & Robins, 2006). If replicated, these findings may suggest that the reduced likelihood of experiencing guilt found among parents may limit their motivation to change their behavior and utilize adaptive conflict resolution strategies, thereby increasing risk for future perpetration. Although speculative, these findings may also suggest that IPV intervention and prevention programs may benefit from assessing and addressing moral emotions (including guilt), particularly among perpetrators who are parents.

Future studies incorporating measures of multiple distressing emotional states, parenting stress, and child age(s) and residential status could inform questions regarding directionality and mechanisms, as well as to determine whether the observed results are specific to guilt or reflective of a general phenomenon of avoiding distressing emotions. Studies employing longitudinal designs are also needed to explore these conceptualizations. Development of measures that assess moral emotions and cognitions regarding one's perpetration of IPV are also needed, as no such measures exist to date. In the current study, the moral guilt subscale assessed the individual's overall moral beliefs (e.g., having a strong sense of right and wrong), but this was not anchored to IPV perpetration or other transgressions. The moral guilt subscale was not correlated with the state or trait subscales for either gender, which suggests that this scale is measuring a unique construct. Measures that more clearly differentiate actions perpetrated vs. experienced and moral cognitions vs. emotions may expand the current research.

Several limitations of this study bear note. The study design would be greatly improved if we were able to longitudinally address the proposed research questions. With the current data, there are also several measurement considerations that may have influenced results, including that all measures were self-report. In particular, we were able to assess an important moral emotion, but this was not assessed with respect to the same timeframe as IPV, nor was the guilt assessment directly anchored to guilt about IPV. In addition, we were not able to directly measure other concepts that may impact guilt, such as life stress and difficulties regulating emotions specifically related to IPV. Additionally, we were not able to assess the ages and cohabitating status of participants' children, likely adding a degree of error to the models, particularly for parents. That is, the parent group may include some individuals with adult children, thus making them more closely resemble the non-parent group. This pattern of error occurred in a manner that likely makes our test of group differences more conservative than the true difference. Further, the sample size potentially led to insufficient power to address some of the research questions (e.g., testing the three-way interaction of parent status, IPV perpetration, and emotion regulation difficulties on guilt). Finally, the findings represent the experiences of heterosexual, predominantly white couples within a rural to semi-rural context. Thus, the generalizability of the findings should be interpreted with caution and future research is needed to understand the unique experiences of diverse groups. The sample was also recruited based on one partner meeting screening criteria for PTSD, which also limits generalizability. However, rates of PTSD diagnoses were similar among parents and non-parents and, although non-parents had slightly more severe PTSD symptoms than parents, because experiential avoidance is common in PTSD (Seligowski et al., 2015), we would have expected non-parents to exhibit difficulty attending to emotions, but this occurred among parents instead. Thus, the nature of the current sample does not appear to have had an impact on the observed results, but examination of the study questions in more broadly generalizable samples will be important.

Conclusion

This study provides preliminary evidence that suggests important theoretical and empirical considerations for future research pertaining to the emotional consequences of IPV perpetration among parents and non-parents. Although additional research is needed to confirm the results, this study suggests that parents do not exhibit elevations of guilt in association with greater IPV perpetration while non-parents do. Although it is unclear why parents display muted guilt responses, we suggest that this may be due to blunted emotional awareness, which could be impacted by stress and impair effective coping strategies. We suggest these theoretical explanations, yet it is important to note that definitive conclusions would be premature at this time and further research is needed to draw conclusions. However, the emotional experiences among parents and non-parents related to IPV perpetration have been minimally studied to date. Thus, the findings herein present an important new line of inquiry and warrant further theoretical and empirical development to understand these processes, as they may have important implications to inform future intervention efforts.

Ethical standards and informed consent

All procedures followed were in accordance with the ethical standards of the responsible committee on human experimentation [institutional and national] and with the Helsinki Declaration of 1975, as revised in 2000. Informed consent was obtained from all patients for being included in the study.

Disclosure of interest statement

Emily C. Taverna, Devin J. McGuire, and Amy D. Marshall declare that they have no conflicts to report.

Funding

This material is based upon work supported by the National Science Foundation Graduate Research Fellowship Program under Grant No. DGE1255832. Any opinions, findings, and conclusions or recommendations expressed in this material are those of the authors and do not necessarily reflect the views of the National Science Foundation.

References

Ansara, D. L., & Hindin, M. J. (2011). Psychosocial consequences of intimate partner violence for women and men in Canada. *Journal of Interpersonal Violence*, *26*(8), 1628–1645. https://doi.org/10.1177/0886260510370600

American Psychiatric Association (2013). Diagnostic and statistical manual of mental disorders (5th ed.). https://doi.org/10.1176/appi.books.9780890425596

Artz, S., Jackson, M. A., Rossiter, K. R., Nijdam-Jones, A., Géczy, I., & Porteous, S. (2014). A comprehensive review of the literature on the impact of exposure to intimate partner violence for children and youth. *International Journal of Child, Youth and Family Studies*, *5*(4), 493–587. https://doi.org/10.18357/ijcyfs54201413274

Bates, D., Machler, M., Bolker, B. M., & Walker, S. C. (2014). Fitting linear mixed-effects models using lme4.

Baumeister, R. F., Stillwell, A. M., & Heatherton, T. F. (1995). Personal narratives about guilt: Role in action control and interpersonal relationships. *Basic and Applied Social Psychology*, *17*(1), 173–198. https://doi.org/10.1207/s15324834basp1701&2_10

Blake, D. D., Weathers, F. W., Nagy, L. M., Kaloupek, D. G., Gusman, F. D., Charney, D. S., & Keane, T. M. (1995). The development of a clinician-administered PTSD scale. *Journal of Traumatic Stress*, *8*(1), 75–90.

Burman, B., Margolin, G., & John, R. S. (1993). America's angriest home videos: Behavioral contingencies observed in home reenactments of marital conflict. *Journal of Consulting and Clinical Psychology*, *61*(1), 28–39. doi: 10.1037//0022-351481.1.17

Bushman, B. J., Baumeister, R. F., & Phillips, C. M. (2001). Do people aggress to improve their mood? Catharsis beliefs, affect regulation opportunity, and aggressive responding. *Journal of Personality and Social Psychology*, *81*(1), 17–32.

Cho, E., & Allen, T. D. (2012). Relationship between work interference with family and parent–child interactive behavior: Can guilt help? *Journal of Vocational Behavior*, *80*(2), 276–287. https://doi.org/10.1016/j.jvb.2011.12.002

Crandall, A., Deater-Deckard, K., & Riley, A. W. (2015). Maternal emotion and cognitive control capacities and parenting: A conceptual framework. *Developmental Review : DR*, *36*, 105–126.

Deater-Deckard, K. (2008). *Parenting stress*. Yale University Press.

Dennis, P. A., Dennis, N. M., Van Voorhees, E. E., Calhoun, P. S., Dennis, M. F., & Beckham, J. C. (2017). Moral transgression during the Vietnam War: A path analysis of the psychological impact of veterans' involvement in wartime atrocities. *Anxiety, Stress, and Coping*, *30*(2), 188–201. https://doi.org/10.1080/10615806.2016.1230669

Doss, B. D., Rhoades, G. K., Stanley, S. M., & Markman, H. J. (2009). The effect of the transition to parenthood on relationship quality: An 8-Year prospective study. *Journal of Personality and Social Psychology*, *96*(3), 601–619. https://doi.org/10.1037/a0013969

Eckhardt, C. I., Murphy, C. M., Whitaker, D. J., Spunger, J., Dykstra, R., & Woodard, K. (2013). The effectiveness of intervention programs for perpetrators and victims of intimate partner violence. *Partner Abuse*, *4*(2), 197–231.

Eisenberg, N., Cumberland, A., & Spinrad, T. L. (1998). Parental socialization of emotion. *Psychological Inquiry*, *9*(4), 241–273. https://doi.org/10.1207/s15327965pli0904_1

Feinberg, M. E. (2003). The internal structure and ecological context of coparenting: A framework for research and intervention. *Parenting, Science and Practice*, *3*(2), 95–131. https://doi.org/10.1207/S15327922PAR0302_01

Gratz, K. L., & Roemer, L. (2004). Multidimensional assessment of emotion regulation and dysregulation: Development, factor structure, and initial validation of the Difficulties in Emotion Regulation Scale. *Journal of Psychopathology and Behavioral Assessment*, *26*(1), 41–54. https://doi.org/10.1023/B:JOBA.0000007455.08539.94

Gustafsson, H. C., & Cox, M. J., (2016). Intimate partner violence in rural low-income families: Correlates and change in prevalence over the first 5 years of a Child's Life. *Journal of Family Violence*, *31*(1), 49–60. https://doi.org/10.1007/s10896-015-9760-4

Hajal, N. J., & Paley, B. (2020). Parental emotion and emotion regulation: A critical target of study for research and intervention to promote child emotion socialization. *Developmental Psychology*, *56*(3), 403–417. https://doi.org/10.1037/dev0000864

Hobfoll, S. E. (2001). The influence of culture, community, and the nested-self in the stress process: Advancing conservation of resources theory. *Applied Psychology*, *50*(3), 337–369. https://doi.org/10.1111/1464-0597.00062

Jones, W. H., Schratter, A. K., & Kugler, K. (2000). The guilt inventory. *Psychological Reports*, *87*(3 Pt 2), 1039–1012. https://doi.org/10.2466/pr0.2000.87.3f.1039

Langhinrichsen-Rohling, J., Misra, T. A., Selwyn, C., & Rohling, M. L. (2012). Rates of bi-directional versus uni-directional intimate partner violence across samples, sexual orientations, and race/ethnicities: A comprehensive review. *Partner Abuse*, *3*(2), 1–2. https://doi.org/10.1891/1946-6560.3.2.e3

Lawrence, E., Orengo-Aguayo, R., Langer, A., & Brock, R. L. (2012). The impact and consequences of partner abuse on partners. *Partner Abuse*, *3*(4), 406–428. https://doi.org/10.1891/1946-6560.3.4.406

Lawrence, E., Rothman, A. D., Cobb, R. J., Rothman, M. T., & Bradbury, T. N. (2008). Marital satisfaction across the transition to parenthood. *Journal of Family Psychology : JFP : Journal of the Division of Family Psychology of the American Psychological Association (Division 43)*, *22*(1), 41–50. https://doi.org/10.1037/0893-3200.22.1.41

Lawrence, A. E., & Taft, C. T. (2013). Shame, posttraumatic stress disorder, and intimate partner violence perpetration. *Aggression and Violent Behavior*, *18*(2), 191–194. https://doi.org/10.1016/j.avb.2012.10.002

Leckman, J., Feldman, R., Swain, J., Eicher, V., Thompson, N., & Mayes, L. (2004). Primary parental occupations: Circuits, genes, and the crucial role of the environment. *Journal of Neural Transmission*, *111*(7), 753–771. https://doi.org/10.1007/s00702-003-0067-x

Litz, B. T., Stein, N., Delaney, E., Lebowitz, L., Nash, W. P., Silva, C., & Maguen, S. (2009). Moral injury and moral repair in war veterans: A preliminary model and intervention strategy. *Clinical Psychology Review*, *29*(8), 695–706.

Mbilinyi, L. F., Edleson, J. L., Hagemeister, A. K., & Beeman, S. K. (2007). What happens to children when their mothers are battered? Results from a four-city anonymous telephone survey. *Journal of Family Violence*, *22*(5), 309–317. https://doi.org/10.1007/s10896-007-9087-x

McDonald, G., O'Brien, L., & Jackson, D. (2007). Guilt and shame: Experiences of parents of self-harming adolescents. *Journal of Child Health Care : For Professionals Working with Children in the Hospital and Community*, *11*(4), 298–310.

McKinney, C. M., Caetano, R., Ramisetty-Mikler, S., & Nelson, S. (2009). Childhood family violence and perpetration and victimization of intimate partner violence: Findings from a national population-based study of couples. *Annals of Epidemiology*, *19*(1), 25–32. https://doi.org/10.1016/j.annepidem.2008.08.008

McNulty, J. K., & Hellmuth, J. C. (2008). Emotion regulation and intimate partner violence in newlyweds. *Journal of Family Psychology : JFP : journal of the Division of Family Psychology of the American Psychological Association (Division 43)*, *22*(5), 794–797. https://doi.org/10.1037/a0013516

Minuchin, P. (1985). Families and individual development: Provocations from the field of family therapy. *Child Development*, *56*(2), 289–302. https://doi.org/10.2307/1129720

Moffitt, T. E., Caspi, A., Krueger, R. F., Magdol, L., Margolin, G., Silva, P. A., & Sydney, R. (1997). Do partners agree about abuse in their relationship? A psychometric evaluation of interpartner agreement. *Psychological Assessment*, *9*(1), 47–56. https://doi.org/10.1037/1040-3590.9.1.47

Owen, A. E., Thompson, M. P., & Kaslow, N. J. (2006). The mediating role of parenting stress in the relation between intimate partner violence and child adjustment. *Journal of Family Psychology : JFP : journal of the Division of Family Psychology of the American Psychological Association (Division 43)*, *20*(3), 505–513.

Raikes, H. Q., & Thompson, R. A. (2005). Efficacy and social support as predictors of parenting stress among families in poverty. *Infant Mental Health Journal*, *26*(3), 177–190.

Rhodes, K. V., Cerulli, C., Dichter, M. E., Kothari, C. L., & Barg, F. K. (2010). I didn't want to put them through that": The influence of children on victim-decision-making in intimate partner violence cases. *Journal of Family Violence*, *25*(5), 485–493. https://doi.org/10.1007/s10896-010-9310-z

Richert, T., Johnson, B., & Svensson, B. (2018). Being a parent to an adult child with drug problems: Negative impacts on life situation, health, and emotions. *Journal of Family Issues*, *39*(8), 2311–2335. https://doi.org/10.1177/0192513X17748695

Rothman, E. F., Mandel, D. G., & Silverman, J. G. (2007). Abusers' perceptions of the effect of their intimate partner violence on children. *Violence against Women*, *13*(11), 1179–1191.

Rutherford, H. J. V., Wallace, N. S., Laurent, H. K., & Mayes, L. C. (2015). Emotion regulation in parenthood. *Developmental Review : DR*, *36*, 1–14.

Salisbury, E. J., Henning, K., & Holdford, R. (2009). Fathering by partner-abusive men: Attitudes on children's exposure to interpersonal conflict and risk factors for child abuse. *Child Maltreatment*, *14*(3), 232–242. https://doi.org/10.1177/1077559509338407

Seligowski, A. V., Lee, D. J., Bardeen, J. R., & Orcutt, H. K. (2015). Emotion regulation and posttraumatic stress symptoms: A meta-analysis. *Cognitive Behaviour Therapy*, *44*(2), 87–102. https://doi.org/10.1080/16506073.2014.980753

Slep, A. M. S., & O'Leary, S. G. (2005). Parent and partner violence in families with young children: Rates, patterns, and connections. *Journal of Consulting and Clinical Psychology*, *73*(3), 435–444. https://doi.org/10.1037/0022-006X.73.3.435

Slobodin, O., Cohen, R., Arden, A., & Katz, I. (2020). Mothers' Need frustration and controlling parenting: The moderating role of maternal guilt. *Journal of Child and Family Studies*, *29*(7), 1914–1926. https://doi.org/10.1007/s10826-020-01720-6

Spencer, C., Mallory, A. B., Cafferky, B. M., Kimmes, J. G., Beck, A. R., & Stith, S. M. (2019). Mental health factors and intimate partner violence perpetration and victimization: A meta-analysis. *Psychology of Violence*, *9*(1), 1–17. https://doi.org/10.1037/vio0000156

Straus, M. A., Hamby, S. L., Boney-McCoy, S., & Sugarman, D. B. (1996). The revised conflict tactics scales (CTS2) development and preliminary psychometric data. *Journal of Family Issues*, *17*(3), 283–316. https://doi.org/10.1177/019251396017003001

Tangney, J. P., Stuewig, J., & Hafez, L. (2011). Shame, guilt and remorse: Implications for offender populations. *The Journal of Forensic Psychiatry & Psychology*, *22*(5), 706–723. https://doi.org/10.1080/14789949.2011.617541

Testa, M., Quigley, B. M., & Leonard, K. E. (2003). Does alcohol make a difference? Within-participants comparison of incidents of partner violence. *Journal of Interpersonal Violence*, *18*(7), 735–743.

Tracy, J. L., & Robins, R. W. (2006). Appraisal antecedents of shame and guilt: Support for a theoretical model. *Personality & Social Psychology Bulletin*, *32*(10), 1339–1351. https://doi.org/10.1177/0146167206290212

Vega, E. M., & O'Leary, K. D. (2007). Test-retest reliability of the Revised Conflict Tactics Scales (CTS2). *Journal of Family Violence, 22*(8), 703–708. https://doi.org/10.1007/s10896-007-9118-7

Weathers, F., Litz, B., Herman, D., Huska, J., & Keane, T. (1993, October). *The PTSD Checklist (PCL): Reliability, Validity, and Diagnostic Utility*. Paper presented at the Annual Convention of the International Society for Traumatic Stress Studies, San Antonio, TX.

OPEN ACCESS

The Trouble with Harman and Lorandos' *Parental Alienation Allegations in Family Court* Study (2020)

Joan S. Meier, Sean Dickson, Chris S. O'Sullivan and Leora N. Rosen

ABSTRACT
Harman and Lorandos assert that they have produced a study analyzing custody cases involving alienation allegations, which "disconfirms" the findings from our study of family court outcomes in cases involving abuse and alienation. In addition to pointing out the authors' misrepresentation and mis-reporting of some of their findings, this Response details a series of profound flaws in their study's design, dataset construction and variable coding, interpretations and analytic approach, as well as a series of statistical errors. The statistical analyses demonstrate that Harman and Lorandos' five findings of a gender bias in favor of fathers are not supported by their data; the only statistically significant findings that persist after re-analysis of the correct data are consistent with the Meier et al. study. These pervasive design and methodological errors undermine both the appearance and assertion of rigor in their approach; these problems and the foundational differences in their dataset from our own disqualify their study from serving as any kind of credible test or disconfirmation of our study.

In 2019, Meier et al. posted online the required final report ("final summary overview") on their 5-year National Institute of Justice (NIJ)-funded study, *Outcomes in Cases Involving Abuse and Alienation Allegations* (Meier et al., 2019; hereafter "FCO study"). In 2020, Meier published an article reporting key portions of the study in a peer-reviewed journal (Meier, 2020). As reported in those two publications, the quantitative findings of the FCO study were consistent with widespread reports that family courts adjudicating custody display patterns of decisions that lead to mothers having reduced or no custody, even when the father is allegedly abusive (Araji & Bosek, 2010; Bemiller, 2008; Berg, 2011; Silberg & Dallam, 2019; Stark et al., 2019). We found that courts frequently reject mothers' claims of fathers' abuse of themselves and their children and that the courts often remove custody from mothers alleging abuse and award it to allegedly abusive fathers. The results we reported in these two publications showed accused fathers' alienation claims exacerbate these outcomes. (While lacking any universal or scientific definition, "parental alienation" or "alienation" is generally understood to refer to one parent's undermining of the children's relationship with the other parent.) Most of the FCO study's hypotheses and findings focused on court responses to abuse and alienation allegations. In limited instances, we also were able to look at effects of gender on court outcomes and found some evidence of gender bias, as well as some similarities in mothers' and fathers' outcomes (Meier et al., 2019, pp. 18-19).

Jennifer Harman and Demosthenes Lorandos assert in a 2021 article entitled *Allegations of Family Violence in Court: How Parental Alienation Affects Judicial Outcomes,* that the Meier et al. study is seriously flawed, and that their own study provides a "direct and thorough test" of its findings, which it "disconfirms" (Harman & Lorandos, 2021, pp. 185, 186, 191, 205). We rebut their critiques of the FCO study's methods in a forthcoming paper (Meier et al., 2022, J. Fam. Ther., Ch. Cust. & Ch. Dev.). Here, we focus instead on Harman and Lorandos' claims about their own study. We will point out multiple serious problems in their methods and analytic strategies, and in their interpretation of their findings and conclusions. We will provide both qualitative and statistical analyses of some of the core errors in their study design, dataset construction and variable coding, interpretations and analytic approach. Our discussion refutes the suggestion that their results "soundly disconfirmed nearly all the findings [they] tested from Meier et al. (2019) report or discovered the findings to be in the opposite direction" (Harman & Lorandos, 2021, p. 22). We conclude by noting the risk that technical jargon, a deluge of statistical and technical detail, and the invocation of transparency (in the form of postings on the Open Science Framework) can mislead readers and reviewers into assuming the scientific validity of a published study that is actually deeply flawed.

Background on Meier, Dickson, Rosen, O'Sullivan & Hayes study

The FCO Study sought to provide an empirical test of widespread criticisms of family courts for their responses to women's abuse reports, found in an extensive qualitative literature (e.g., Jaffe et al., 2003; Silberg et al., 2013; Smith & Coukos, 1997; Stark et al., 2019); small quantitative studies (Silberg & Dallam, 2019; Berg, 2011; Bemiller, 2008; California Protective Parents Association, 2018) and widespread public reports on social media and elsewhere (*One Mom's Battle,* 2021; *The Court Said*, 2021). These critics describe a resistant and sometimes hostile response from family courts to mothers' reports of family abuse; the use of parental alienation claims by allegedly abusive fathers to defeat mothers' abuse allegations; courts' awards of unsupervised access and custody to allegedly abusive fathers; and particularly negative responses to mothers' and children's child sexual abuse allegations.

Building on a small pilot study of alienation cases (Meier & Dickson, 2017), the FCO Study proposed to expand Meier and Dickson's innovative approach to gathering data on family court practices: retrieving and analyzing electronically published decisions from across US custody courts to obtain a national picture of such courts' behavior. The National Institute of Justice (NIJ) funded the study. Law graduates were employed to "search for all electronically published decisions in the U.S. in which there were allegations of both abuse and parental alienation, allegations of abuse but not alienation, and allegations of alienation but not abuse" (Meier et al., 2014). The coders simply entered into a database the types of allegations, other case information, and court outcomes.

The reported findings are straightforward, consisting primarily of frequencies or percentages of different outcomes in different categories of cases. The Study found that courts reject mothers' claims of abuse more often than not, and that mothers' claims that the father abused the child are associated with more frequent losses of custody. Fathers' claims that mothers alienated the child are associated with an increase in courts' disbelief in mothers' abuse claims and an increase in their loss of custody. We also reported some findings that support assertions by alienation theory proponents (Meier, 2020; Meier et al., 2019).

Harman and Lorandos' study does not test, replicate or disconfirm Meier et al.'s findings

Harman & Lorandos acknowledge that Meier et al.'s search string and User Manual were publicly posted months before they published their study. They chose not to replicate the study's method, apparently deeming the large dataset unmanageable (Harman & Lorandos, 2021, p. 7, note 3). Harman and Lorandos assert that the fact that they did not literally replicate our methods nor use our data is not a problem because their study, "as designed, provides a stronger and more transparent test of the [Meier et al.] hypotheses" (Harman & Lorandos, 2021, p. 192). We explain their study was neither strong nor transparent, and that its design made testing Meier et al.'s hypotheses or findings impossible.

We will discuss Harman and Lorandos' article's misrepresentation of the data they posted on OSF, as well as their representation of findings they knew were incorrect. We discuss why their study could not test the FCO study's findings and analyze key methodological (non-statistical) flaws in their approach, which cast doubt on many of their findings. Lastly, we focus on the statistical errors that compound these design flaws and further impugn their findings.

Miscoded data and suppression of corrected results

Harman and Lorandos acknowledge in a footnote that at some point they discovered a pattern of mis-coded data in their dataset: Numerous cases in which the court determined parental alienation occurred or did not occur had not been "originally classified in that way" (p. 196, note 5). After correcting the mis-codes, they state that they analyzed their hypotheses again and posted the output on the Open Science Framework. The article then reports that the "research results were similar to those presented in this article; however, the effects were often stronger (see footnote 1)" (Harman & Lorandos, 196, n. 5). An examination of their postings on Open Science Framework reveals this description to be false and misleading.

Over the course of their paper, Harman and Lorandos report five purportedly significant regression results showing that fathers accused of alienation are more likely to lose custody or parenting time than mothers so accused (Harman & Lorandos, 2021, pp. 197-98, 199, 200, 202). As shown in Table 1 below, however, every one of these findings is *not* significant according to the authors' *own regression analyses of the corrected data posted on OSF*. Harman and Lorandos' core gender finding – that fathers accused of alienation are more likely to lose custody of their children than mothers so accused – is an artifact of their miscoded data.

For instance, Harman and Lorandos assert in their analysis of Hypothesis 1 "that fathers had 1.73 greater odds (63.30% greater likelihood) of losing custody of their child(ren) than did mothers ($p = .002$)" (Harman & Lorandos, 2021, pp 197-98). Yet, in their posted analysis of the corrected data, the effect is smaller (OR 1.55) and not significant: $p = 0.053$ (Harman & Lorandos OSF, 2020, *Analyses, CourtDetermined PA or not as predictor, Hypothesis 1*) (see Table 1). Similarly, the authors assert under Hypothesis 1a that fathers are more likely to lose custody to abusive mothers than the reverse: OR 2.33, $p = 0.037$ (p. 200), claiming this finding is "opposite … the one that Meier et al. reported" (p. 204). Yet their posted corrected odds ratio suggests mothers lose custody more often than fathers (OR = 0.15), though the difference is not significant (Table 1, $p = 0.999$; Harman & Lorandos OSF 2020, *Analyses, CourtDetermined PA or not as predictor, Hypothesis 1a*). And last, in their Hypothesis 6 findings, Harman and Lorandos assert that "alienated fathers had almost 6 times the odds (85.67%

Table 1. Differences in effect size and significance of independent variables in subsets of Harman and Lorandos' hypotheses 1, 1a, 3, and 6, using reported data with coding mistakes and unreported data with coding corrections.

	Hypothesis 1 – Outcomes Overall, without Accounting for Abuse Claims				Hypothesis 1a – Outcomes in Founded Abuse Cases				Hypothesis 3 – Outcomes when Alienating Parent Alleges Abuse			
	Alienated Parent Lost Custody				Alienated Parent Lost Custody				Alienated Parent Lost Custody			
	Reported (miscoded data)		On OSF (corrected data)		Reported (miscoded data)		On OSF (corrected data)		Reported (miscoded data)		On OSF (corrected data)	
Predictor	Odds Ratio	*p*	Odds Ratio	*p*	Odds Ratio	*p*	Odds Ratio	*p*	Odds Ratio	*p*	Odds Ratio	*p*
Gender	1.725	0.002	1.549	0.053*	2.331	0.037	0.015	0.999*	1.6	0.048	1.537	0.171*
Alienation Founded	2.406	<0.001	3.824	<0.001	2.445	0.028	387.799	0.999*	2.823	<0.001	4.157	<0.001
Interaction term	1.2	0.296	1.074	0.752	1.238	0.599	163.875	0.999	1.277	0.302	0.986	0.964
Reported N	953^				122^				386^			
Actual N	189		162		48		35		108		91	

	Hypothesis 6 – Outcome for Alienated Parent, Considering Count of Unfounded Abuse Claims							
	Alienated Parent Lost Parenting Time				Alienated Parent Lost Custody			
	Reported (miscoded data)		On OSF (corrected data)		Reported (miscoded data)		On OSF (corrected data)	
Predictor	Odds Ratio	*p*	Odds Ratio	*p*	Odds Ratio	*p*	Odds Ratio	*p*
Count of Unfounded Abuse Allegations	0.564	0.022	0.612	0.064*	0.845	0.204	0.943	0.758
Gender	5.98	0.031	3.196	0.181*	0.547	0.036	0.675	0.223*
Alienation Founded	10.08	<0.001	23.536	<0.001	0.396	0.001	0.294	<0.001
Interaction term	0.661	0.097	0.68	0.146	0.969	0.808	1.094	0.628
Reported N	348				NR			
Actual N	348		292		93		79	

* Change in significance with corrected data. ^ Number of cases was misreported. Corrected data refers to analyses performed by Harman and Lorandos using their own corrections to the data; these analyses were posted on Open Science Foundation (OSF) but were not included in the manuscript. In the reported data, N was reported as the number of cases submitted to the model; "Actual N" is the number of cases included in the model after missing data were dropped.

Table 2. Comparison of frequency of alienation founding by gender in Harman and Lorandos' uncorrected, reported data and corrected, unreported data.

Reported Data, with Coding Mistakes		Unreported Data, with Coding Corrections					
		Father Accused of Alienation			% Incorrectly Coded in Original Regression	Not Addressed	Grand Total
		Alleged	Founded	Total			
Father Accused of Alienation	Alleged	86	55*	141	39%	72	213
	Founded	17*	215	231	7%	13	245
	Total	103	270	373	19%	85	458
		Mother Accused of Alienation					
Mother Accused of Alienation	Alleged	120	44*	164	27%	84	248
	Founded	24*	206	230	10%	17	247
	Total	144	250	394	17%	101	495

* Cells with coding mistakes in reported data. Corrected data refers to analyses performed by Harman and Lorandos using their own corrections to the data; these analyses were posted on Open Science Foundation (OSF) but were not included in the manuscript. In the data reported in the manuscript, N represents the number of cases in the model; "Actual N" is the number of cases included in the model after missing data were dropped.

greater likelihood) of mothers of getting a decrease in custody than did alienated mothers (p = .031)" (p. 202). In their corrected data, though, this effect drops to odds of 3.20 and is not significant (Table 1, p = 0.181; Harman & Lorandos OSF, 2020, *Analyses, CourtDetermined PA or not as predictor, Hypothesis 6*).

In short, Harman and Lorandos' core gender finding - that fathers accused of alienation are more likely to lose custody of their children than mothers so accused - is simply an artifact of their miscoded data, which is seen in the authors' own *posted but unreported* analyses.

Based on Harman and Lorandos' own analyses of their corrected data posted on OSF, the only significant gender effects that remain significant with their corrected data are (i) that mothers accused of alienation are more likely to lose their case than fathers so accused (Hypothesis 1; corrected data OR 0.68, p = 0.001), and (ii) that courts are less likely to credit mothers' abuse allegations than fathers': Hypothesis 2; corrected data Beta −0.20, p = 0.004 (Harman & Lorandos OSF 2020, *Analyses, Found or Alleged as Predictor, Hypothesis 1, 2*; also shown in Tables 1 and 2 below). Both of these findings are consistent with and not "in the opposite direction" (Harman & Lorandos, 2021, pp. 204) of Meier et al.'s findings (*see generally* Meier et al., 2019, p. 18; Meier, 2020, p. 100). Both results indicate that courts disfavor mothers, as we found, not fathers, as they claim to have found.

Oddly, Harman and Lorandos acknowledge in a later footnote (note 7, p. 200) that they did not find gender effects in a separate set of analyses which they characterize as based only on whether or not the court found parental alienation. However, such a variable is not described elsewhere in the paper - and there were only two sets of analyses posted on the

Open Science Framework. If the authors were referring to the second (corrected) analyses on OSF, footnote 7 appears to directly contradict their claim in footnote 5 that the corrected analyses show similar or stronger gender effects.

Further examination reveals why Harman and Lorandos incorrectly found bias against fathers: Their coding errors themselves were systematically biased by gender. As shown in Table 2 below (constructed from Harman and Lorandos' own postings on OSF), the corrected data indicate that at least 39% of fathers' cases were erroneously coded as alleged rather than founded alienation; yet only 27% of mothers' cases were so miscoded. Harman and Lorandos' posted data show that nearly 1 in 5 cases (18%, 140/767) in their data were miscoded. They do not report the extent of this miscoding in the article, and only reference the issue obliquely in the footnote quoted above. The original coding incorrectly coded alienation allegations against fathers as unfounded 46% more often than mothers (RR 1.46, $p=0.032$). This produced Harman and Lorandos' finding of bias against fathers in the courts, mistaking the impact of founded alienation for a gender effect.

Non-statistical methodological flaws

In numerous respects, key codes in the authors' study appear to be internally contradictory or erroneous, with important implications for the accuracy of their tests of their own data. In addition, several of their assertions about their findings are inaccurate.

Problem 1: Harman and Lorandos' dataset is both too narrow and too heterogeneous to produce any useful findings or to test the FCO study findings

Too narrow

The FCO study specifically included abuse cases with and without alienation claims, in order to compare them. Harman and Lorandos' dataset consists solely of alienation cases; they have no abuse cases without alienation claims. Consequently, their dataset cannot test the impact of claims of alienation on court outcomes for parents alleging abuse relative to cases *without* alienation claims.

Too heterogeneous

Harman and Lorandos included every possible sort of case referencing alienation, whether it was a private custody case or a case filed by the state (e.g., for child neglect), a case in which both parents claimed the other was abusive, or a case occasioned by relocation, incarceration, or any other issue. Harman and Lorandos criticize the FCO study's deliberate exclusion of such cases (Harman & Lorandos, 2021, p. 186), but the FCO study was explicitly focused on *custody litigation between parents* precisely because that is where the field's controversies over abuse and alienation have arisen, and where the particular gender dynamics of mothers vs. fathers are found. Alienation claims are designed for use against an opposing parent, not the State. State cases, in contrast, are not comparing two parents but determining whether children should be removed altogether, often due to neglect by one or both parents. In addition, State abuse and neglect cases are governed by restrictive standards for "substantiation" or "founding" of allegations – these standards are entirely different from custody courts' determinations (by a preponderance of evidence) of allegations of abuse and alienation (Kornblum & Pollack, 2018). These cases are not comparable to parent vs. parent custody battles over abuse and alienation claims, and their inclusion unavoidably compromises any conclusions that may be drawn about custody courts' responses to parents' alienation and/or abuse claims.

The problem with Harman and Lorandos' mixing State and non-State cases can be seen vividly in their definition of their "custody loss" variable – which includes state terminations of parental rights (Harman & Lorandos, 2021, p. 196). In their study, State removals of children into foster care, and even termination of all parental rights, are treated as equivalent to one parent losing primary parenting or most visitation in favor of the other parent.

Another problem with the inclusion of State cases is their equating of neglect allegations with "abuse" (Harman & Lorandos, 2021, p. 194). Neglect claims are common in State cases, but, in our experience, are seldom raised in private custody litigation. "Neglect" typically lacks a clear, objective definition, particularly in child custody statutes. That is why the FCO study excluded them from its definition of abuse (Meier, 2019, App. A, p. 1). State findings of parental neglect, typically addressing failure to feed and/or clothe, get them to school, etc., cannot be compared to the physical or sexual abuse allegations against which alienation cross claims are often brought to bear. In short, inclusion of State-initiated neglect claims in the dataset makes it impossible to draw any conclusions from this dataset about how custody courts addressing alienation respond to actual abuse claims by a parent.

Additional categorization and coding confusions further muddy the waters of Harman and Lorandos' study. Not only do the authors treat a switch of primary parenting from one party to the other the same as a

State termination of parental rights, they also bring into the "loss of custody" category significant limitations of visitation time (Harman & Lorandos, 2021, p. 196). A reduction in visitation or a switch to supervised visitation with one's child is not comparable to a loss of primary custody, nor to a complete termination of all parental rights. Only four cases were coded in this way, but the decision to code termination of parental rights in two contradictory ways – both as a loss of custody for both parents and as reduced parenting time for one parent –making the findings difficult to interpret on their own, and impossible to compare to ours. Review of their postings reveals that Harman and Lorandos include cases in which *both* parents' parental rights were terminated in their analysis of rates at which alienating parents lost parenting time (Harman & Lorandos OSF, 2020), further obscuring the meaning of their results. The FCO study carefully defined loss of custody to mean loss of primary care of the children in favor of the other parent (Meier et al., 2019, p. 8).

Harman and Lorandos extoll their decision to include every possible type of case, including mutual abuse cases, in their dataset as a means of increasing "external validity" (Harman & Lorandos, 2021, p. 186). Yet the inclusion of not only State cases, but also cases with mutual abuse claims, or where a parent accused of alienation was also accused of abuse, unavoidably confounds their conclusions. Such cases are not comparable to cases where one parent alleges abuse and the other alienation; in the more complex ones, it is impossible to know which allegations drove a court's decision. Rather than increasing "external validity," then, Harman and Lorandos' failure to exclude or control for cases with mutual abuse claims or co-occurring abuse and alienation claims in their regression analysis *decreases* the validity of their findings because they have conflated cases in which an alienating parent lost custody *due to abuse* with those in which that parent might well have lost custody due to alienation.

Harman and Lorandos' data posted on OSF indicate that only 25% of mothers accused of alienation were simultaneously accused of abuse (124/495), but 38% of fathers were accused of both (176/458), i.e., fathers were 53% more likely than mothers to be accused of both abuse and alienation (RR 1.53, CI 1.21-1.95, $p < 0.001$; Meier et al., 2021, p. 26). If courts were likely to remove children from parents accused of both alienation and abuse more often than parents accused of just alienation, this would be obscured by the authors' characterization of both types of cases as custody losses for fathers "accused of alienation." (Harman & Lorandos, 2021, pp. 199, 200, 202). In short, both the study's exclusions and inclusions render their findings uninterpretable, and their conclusions likely wrong.

Problem 2: Conflating trial court and appellate decisions in coding outcomes

Because the FCO Study's goal was to examine the decision-making of trial courts, which are responsible for evaluating evidence and issuing discretionary decisions about custody and access, that study focused solely on trial court decisions, although it used both trial and appellate opinions as the source of that information (Meier, 2019 App. B, p. 1). In contrast, although their paper is opaque on this point, Harman and Lorandos appear to have coded appellate and trial court determinations interchangeably. For example, they write that the loss of custody "had to occur or be affirmed at the end of the appellate decision" (Harman & Lorandos, 2021, p. 194), and refer to reductions in parenting time "after the trial-level and appeals process" (Harman & Lorandos, 2021, p. 196). Review of their dataset on OSF confirms that they coded custody losses only if the appeals court affirmed them; they coded no custody loss if the appeals court reversed such a ruling (Harman & Lorandos, 2020, OSF, *Data and Process Notes*). They also assert that their "findings indicate that *appellate* courts do not take all claims of alienation or domestic violence or child abuse at face value. These claims are evaluated based on the evidence presented" (Harman & Lorandos, 2021, p. 23; emphasis added).

This last statement evinces a fundamental misconception about appellate process. Appellate courts do not "evaluate the evidence" like trial courts. Nor do appellate courts determine whether abuse or alienation claims are valid as all first-year law students learn. Unlike trial courts, which take testimony and admit evidence, appellate courts do none of that: They are limited to reviewing the written record to determine if the trial court properly *interpreted the law* and used the correct *procedures* when considering the case (Council of California, 2021). An appellate court could thus (in theory) agree with a trial court's factual finding of abuse or alienation and also agree with a decision not to change custody, but still be compelled to reverse the decision on other legal or procedural grounds. Treating such a procedural reversal as a "loss of custody" is fundamentally erroneous - because appeals courts do not exercise discretion to determine custody, as do trial courts. Rather, appeals court reversals typically simply tell trial courts they did something procedurally or legally wrong, usually resulting in a remand to the trial court to re-decide. Appeals court reversals (or affirmances) thus have no bearing on the substantive questions driving both studies: how *fact-finding* and discretion-exercising courts treat abuse and alienation allegations when deciding custody. By conflating appellate and trial court outcomes, the study makes it impossible to discern how courts are applying their discretion to the facts and claims, the question both studies seek to answer.

Table 3. Comparison of Harman and Lorandos' original coding of custody loss and re-coding for regression analysis.

	Harman and Lorandos' Re-Coding of Custody Loss for Regression						
	Mother Accused of Alienation			Father Accused of Alienation			
	Custody Loss			Custody Loss			
Original Custody Loss Coding	No	Yes	Missing	No	Yes	Missing	Total
No Custody Loss	0	0	394*	1	0	367*	762*
Mother Lost Custody	0	50	0	22	0	0	191
Father Lost Custody	49	0	0	0	67	0	
Other Party Lost Custody	0	0	2*	0	0	1*	3*

*Cases were improperly coded as "Missing" instead of "No Custody Loss" for regression analysis.

Another legal confusion appears in the authors' reference to family courts' findings of "guilty" or "not guilty." These terms and concepts do not apply in custody litigation, but only to criminal prosecution (Harman & Lorandos, 2021, p. 208 Table A2, p. 195 Table 3).

Problem 3. Additional problem with custody loss variable

Harman and Lorandos' definition of "Total Loss of Custody" includes awards of extremely limited supervised visits. They offer no rationale for this decision (Harman & Lorandos, 2021, p. 194). Cases coded as "custody losses" thus include the following examples, among others: "Father's visitation [was] cut down to four hours of supervised visitation every other weekend," "Father was given limited supervision with his son," and "Mother's petition to relocate granted. Father allowed continued supervised visitation" (Harman & Lorandos OSF, 2020, Cases 547, 597, 631). In some of these cases, fathers only had visitation to begin with, yet these outcomes are still coded as a "total loss of custody." As far as we can tell from a review of the coding notes, these codings appear for fathers but *not* for mothers in the study's dataset. The net effect is that mothers' actual losses of primary custody are equated with fathers' visitation *reductions* or unchanged restrictions, creating a systemic gender bias.

Problem 4. Treating professional opinions as equivalent to court opinions in defining "founded" alienation

The FCO Study explicitly set out to analyze *court* rulings, defining "crediting" of alienation and abuse allegations to mean judicial findings or the equivalent, i.e., party admissions or criminal convictions for abuse (Meier, 2020, 103 note 8; User Guide, Appendix B). Harman and Lorandos code alienation as "founded" if *either* a judge *or* a neutral appointee (custody evaluator or guardian ad litem) believed a parent had alienated a child from the other parent (Harman & Lorandos, 2021, pp. 194, 200-201). They treat alienation as "founded" even when the court *disagreed* with the appointed professional on that point (Harman & Lorandos, 2021, p. 194). But when a court disagrees with a professional's testimony, it is the court's finding that drives the court's decision. There are a number of important statistical tests that could have been affected by this problematic coding decision. For instance, both their Hypotheses 1 and 1a address the impact of "founded" alienation on court outcomes (Harman & Lorandos, 2021, pp. 197-199), yet their analysis includes cases where the court did *not* find alienation.

A similar problem may be embedded in Harman and Lorandos' discussion of "founded" abuse (Harman & Lorandos, 2021, p. 194). As with alienation, the authors speak of coding allegations as founded or not based on decisions of *either* "investigators or the court" (Harman & Lorandos, 2021, p. 196). They refer to abuse allegations in terms that reflect outside evaluations, not court findings: They code them as "substantiated" or "unsubstantiated," "false" or "unknown" after an "investigation" (Harman & Lorandos, 2021, Appendix A2). "Investigation" is a term used for evaluators, not courts' fact-finding. The authors also remark that a finding of abuse can be based on "something as little as an "inarticulable hunch" of a CPS caseworker" (Harman & Lorandos, 2021, p. 194). They also describe "founded" abuse as a "highly discretionary and unconstrained conclusion drawn by investigators," without mentioning courts' concurrence or lack thereof (Harman & Lorandos, 2021, p. 205). It appears that they have deemed abuse claims founded or unfounded based on the results of outside "investigations" by evaluators or agencies, as well as by courts. Therefore, it seems possible that, as in their handling of alienation, they coded as "unfounded" abuse allegations that were deemed unfounded by outside evaluators or "investigators," *even if the courts, after hearing more evidence, deemed them credible.* If so, it would help to explain their odd conclusion that courts award *more* parenting time to parents who make allegations coded as false, and less parenting time to parents subject to "unfounded" accusations (Harman & Lorandos, 2021, p. 202). They call such unfounded claims a "silver bullet" strategy that rewards the parent making false accusations (Harman & Lorandos, 2021, p. 205). Given the illogic and unlikelihood of such an outcome, we wonder if those cases they describe as "rewarding false claims" actually involved abuse allegations coded as "unfounded" by an outside investigator but validated by the *court.*

Problem 5. Inapplicable evaluator/GAL analysis (Harman & Lorandos hypothesis 4)

Harman and Lorandos assert that their analysis of the impact of court-appointed professionals on mothers' vs. fathers' outcomes undermines faith in Meier et al.'s finding that the presence of court-appointed neutral professionals, i.e., Guardians Ad Litem (GALs) or custody evaluators, significantly disfavors mothers (Harman & Lorandos, 2021, pp. 200-201; Meier et al., 2019, pp. 21-23). But the FCO study compared cases with these professionals to those without: Harman and Lorandos simply compare mothers' vs. fathers' outcomes in cases with these professionals and find no difference. This finding offers the surface appearance of gender equality but says little about true gender equity because that would depend at minimum on whether the mothers' and fathers' cases involve comparable facts and postures.

Harman and Lorandos contradict themselves regarding which cases they actually analyzed when they were looking at the effects of professionals testifying. They state at one point that their analysis was restricted to cases in which a custody evaluator or GAL made a finding of alienation (Harman & Lorandos, 2021, p. 200), but then state that the finding of no gender difference in outcomes applies "whether they were found to be alienating parents or not" (Harman & Lorandos, 2021, p. 201). If they did limit the analysis to "founded" alienation, such an analysis is of questionable meaning and has no bearing on the FCO study's finding.

Problem 6. Apparent misinterpretation of own finding

Harman and Lorandos' Hypothesis 2 reads as follows: "When a mother claims intrafamilial abuse and the father claims PA, her reports of abuse will be deemed unfounded more often than if the father claimed abuse and the mother claimed PA" (Harman & Lorandos, 2021, p. 199). This hypothesis, while not identical to ours, does parallel one of the FCO study's gender-specific findings. We found that when a mother accused a father of abuse and he accused her of alienation, outcomes for mothers were significantly worse than if he did not make the alienation claim; the same was not true for fathers when they alleged abuse by the mother and the mother accused them of alienation (Meier et al., 2019, pp. 18-19, 22-23).

Harman and Lorandos conclude that they "did not find support for Hypothesis 2," because "fathers were more likely than mothers to have unfounded allegations of abuse made about them" (Harman & Lorandos, 2021, p. 200). This statement actually *confirms their hypothesis* that mothers' abuse allegations are "deemed unfounded" more often than fathers'. That is, if allegations against fathers are more often "unfounded" than allegations against mothers, this means that *courts disbelieve mothers' abuse allegations more often than fathers' abuse allegations.* We can only surmise that Harman and Lorandos' failure to understand their own verbiage reflects their confirmation bias and determination to disprove the FCO Study's findings and others' critiques of court biases against mothers. An objective reading of *their own words* compels recognition that their finding is actually *consistent with* both the FCO Study's findings and the abuse field's critique.

Problem 7. Additional concordant findings denied

Harman and Lorandos fail to acknowledge the apparent convergence of at least two more of their findings with the FCO study's. In their analyses of Hypotheses 1 and 1a, they conclude that parents found to be alienating are more likely to lose custody or parenting time, regardless of gender. They cite this finding as "fail[ing] to...support the conclusions made by Meier et al." (Harman & Lorandos, 2021, p. 183). Yet the FCO study produced virtually the same finding (Meier et al., 2019, p. 18). Their finding related to Hypothesis 1a is also consistent with the FCO Study (Meier et al., 2019, p. 17). Both concluded that even "founded" abuse is sometimes outweighed by findings of alienation (Meier et al., 2019, pp. 15, 18). It is hard to understand Harman and Lorandos' refusal (even after it was pointed out to them, https://osf.io/j9bh5) to recognize that these findings are convergent.

The appearance of bias also arises from Harman and Lorandos' conclusion that "the majority of courts carefully weigh allegations of all forms of family violence" (Harman & Lorandos, 2021, p. 183). This was not a question that was asked or answered in any of their hypotheses or statistical analyses - nor ours. Their assertion is based on a handful of interviews with founded abusers' attorneys (Harman & Lorandos, 2021, pp. 204-205). Such opinions provide no objective assessment, let alone scientifically valid evidence.

Statistical errors

Statistical error 1. Improper interpretation of the effects and significance of key independent variables

In their regression analyses, Harman and Lorandos improperly interpret the effects and significance of their independent variables in two regards: 1) they fail to consider the interaction term when interpreting the effect of gender and alienation as individual covariates, and 2) they interpret the interaction term in their non-linear models as though they had used a linear model. These mistakes cause them to state the effect of key variables incorrectly as well as to improperly test several of their hypotheses which turn on the significance of the interaction term.

Misinterpretation of main effects

In discussing Hypothesis 1, Harman and Lorandos report that they "found a statistically significant gender main effect, such that fathers had 1.73 greater odds (63.30% greater likelihood) of losing their child(ren) than did mothers (p=.002)." Similarly, in regard to alienation they found that, "if there was a known alienating parent, this parent had 2.41:1 greater odds (70.64% greater likelihood) of losing custody of their children than was an alleged alienating parent (p = .002...)" (Harman & Lorandos, 2021, pp. 197-198). Both of these findings are drawn from their regression output for the individual gender and alienation variables. However, their regression model also includes an interaction variable for gender and alienation, which is the gender variable multiplied by the alienation variable. Because the gender and alienation variables are also present in the interaction variable, it is not accurate to report the effect of the individual variables without factoring in their presence in the interaction variable.

In its most simple format, Harman and Lorandos' regression equation for custody loss takes this form (omitting the intercept and error terms for simplicity):

$$\text{Custody Loss} = \beta_1{}^*\text{Gender} + \beta_2{}^*\text{Alienation} + \beta_3{}^*\left(\text{Gender}^*\text{Alienation}\right).$$

In their article, Harman and Lorandos report the parameters for β_1 and β_2 as the effects of gender and alienation (Harman & Lorandos, 2021, p. 98, Table 7), but they have neglected to account for the effect of β_3, causing them to misreport the effect of gender and alienation in the model (Darlington & Hayes (2017, p. 433). Jaccard & Turrisi (2003, p. 24) specifically caution that these coefficients should not be interpreted as main effects, as Harman and Lorandos have done, when there is an interaction variable in the equation.

Moreover, because Harman and Lorandos' model is (necessarily) non-linear, this error cannot be rectified by simply adding the interaction effect (β_3) to report the effect of gender or alienation as in a linear model. In a non-linear model, this addition would have to take place before transforming the regression coefficients into an odds ratio, resulting in an uninterpretable "ratio of ratios." Due to this complexity, *when a non-linear model includes an interaction term, odds ratios are considered an inappropriate means of interpreting the effect of any particular variable* (Karaca-Mandic et al., 2012, pp. 266-267). Rather than interpreting main effects and interactions as though the model were linear, the researcher must estimate *average marginal effects* predicted under the model for the variable of interest, here, gender (Karaca-Mandic et al., 2012, p. 270). We perform this analysis in the final section of this article.

Misinterpretation of interaction term

In addition to misinterpreting the main effects of gender and alienation because they are also present in the interaction term, Harman and Lorandos misinterpret the significance of their gender-alienation interaction term in several of their analyses. They conclude that their Hypothesis 1 is unsupported because the p-value of the interaction term does not reach statistical significance (Harman & Lorandos, 2021, p. 198). Because their model is non-linear, the significance of the interaction term varies at each point on the distribution, which means one cannot interpret the significance of the interaction term based solely on the p-value reported in the regression output, as one would with a linear model. This treatment of a non-linear model as though it were linear is considered a "common mistake" (Buis, 2010, p. 305; Ai & Norton, 2003, p. 129). The appropriate test of significance for an interaction term in a non-linear model is to consider the "difference-in-differences" in the average marginal effects predicted for the interaction of the two variables of interest. We perform this analysis for Hypothesis 1 in the final section of this article.

Statistical error 2. Improper construction of custody loss variable

Compounding the errors in interpreting main effects and interactions, Harman and Lorandos (presumably unintentionally) deviated from their analytic plan when they constructed their custody loss variable for the regression. This error results in over 80% of the cases in their data set being omitted from the analysis, as can be seen in Table 3 below.

The authors' analytic plan states that the dependent variable is coded as "custody loss" if the alleged alienating parent lost all parenting time and "no custody loss" if the parent did not lose all parenting time (Harman & Lorandos, 2021, p. 195, Table 3). Yet, when they construct the custody loss variable for the regression, they instead compare custody losses to custody *gains* by an allegedly alienating parent (rather than to *no custody loss*). Table 3 below compares Harman and Lorandos' original coding of custody loss with their re-coding of the custody loss variable used in the regression analysis.

The dataset posted on OSF contains 953 cases with a coded custody outcome (p. 196) of which 191 cases result in a custody loss and 762 do not result in a custody loss (Harman & Lorandos OSF, 2020, "Data and Process Notes, SPSS cleaned appellate case dataset"). As shown in Table 3 above, only 191 cases with a custody loss are included in the custody loss dependent variable in the regression posted on OSF. Because the regression equation only compares one parent's custody

Table 4. Comparison of effect and standard coding of gender and alienation as predictors of loss of custody in binary logistic regression.

Covariates	Results with Effect Coding (+1/-1)		Results with Standard Coding (1/0)	
	Odds Ratio	p-value	Odds Ratio	p-value
Gender	1.73	0.002	2.07	0.119*
Alienation	2.41	<0.001	4.02	0.001
Interaction Term	1.2	0.296	2.07	0.296
Model Fit Statistics				
N	189		189	
Chi-Sq	39.91		39.91	
Pearson	<0.0001		<0.0001	
Log-Likelihood	−105.64		−105.64	
Pseudo R^2	0.16		0.16	

* Change in significance due to use of "effect coding".

Note: This table shows that the coding change from 0/1 to -1/1 affected the regression output for the Gender, Alienation, and Interaction terms. Harman and Lorandos erroneously did not change their interpretive approach, reporting the results of their regression as though Gender and Alienation were coded as 0/1 rather than as -1/1.

losses to the other parent's custody losses in order to determine in how many cases custody was lost, it leaves out all of the cases where *neither* parent lost custody.

Harman and Lorandos report in their Table 3 an N of 953 for custody loss regression, but regression output on OSF shows that 764 of those cases were not included in the regression, having been omitted and called "missing data." Similar discrepancies are seen between their OSF data and their published article's reports of the Ns for Hypotheses 1a, 3, and 6 (Table 1).

The same error also leads to systematically biased gender findings. The erroneous regression coding of custody loss versus custody gain, rather than custody loss versus no custody loss, overstates the rate at which fathers lost custody relative to mothers. Comparing losses to gains, as Harman and Lorandos did, fathers accused of alienation lose custody 74% (67/89) of the time compared to mothers 51% (50/99) (Table 3). When all the actual cases with no custody loss are included in the regression variable for "no custody loss," as envisioned by the analysis plan, fathers lose custody only 15% of the time (67/457), compared to mothers' loss of custody 10% of the time (50/495) (Table 3). Thus, under erroneous analysis, fathers have 2.98 times greater odds of losing custody than mothers ($p < 0.001$). Corrected analysis reduces these odds by approximately 50%, to 1.53 ($p = 0.041$).

This significant gender effect is a simple effect and does not control for whether alienation was founded, a variable with enormous impact on custody outcomes according to both studies. In Table 4 of their article, Harman and Lorandos report that 72% of fathers compared to 63% of mothers were found to be alienators (Harman & Lorandos, 2021, p. 197). This means that fathers had 1.5 times the odds of mothers of being found to be alienators (p=.01); thus, the significant gender difference in custody loss. After we corrected for Harman and Lorandos' compounded errors,

Table 5. Logistic regression of custody loss, by gender, alienation alleged, alienation found, and interaction; summary statistics and predicted frequency of custody loss (average marginal effects).

Observations			
N = 767	Pseudo R-Squared = 0.06	Log Likelihood -281.98	
Average Marginal Effects – Predicted Custody Loss Frequency in Each Scenario			
Predictor	Margin	Difference	p-value
Mother	11.69%	3.11%	0.194
Father	14.81%		
Alienation Alleged	3.67%	14.07%	<0.001
Alienation Found	17.74%		
Mother, Alienation Alleged	3.47%	12.13%	<0.001
Mother, Alienation Found	15.60%		
Father, Alienation Alleged	3.88%	16.12%	<0.001
Father, Alienation Found	20.00%		
Difference-in-Differences (Mother vs. Father, Alleged vs Found)		3.99%	0.335

we found no significant main or interaction effects involving gender in our regression model. (See section "Re-analysis of part of hypothesis 1 with corrected coding and regression methodology" below).

Statistical error 3. Improper use of "effect coding" for gender and alienation

Harman and Lorandos note that they had originally intended to dummy code the independent variables "Gender of (alleged) Alienator" and "Founded or Alleged PA" as 0/1, but they changed the coding to −1/1 "to compare the two groups with the interaction term" (Harman & Lorandos, 2021, p. 195, Table 3), a technique called 'effect coding' (Hardy, 1993, p. 64). Harman and Lorandos wanted to "compare the two groups with the interaction term" yet they seem to have overlooked the change in dummy coding when interpreting their regression output, rendering their interpretation of the odds ratios incorrect.

"Effect coding" is used when "one wants to contrast subgroups with a sample average," (Hardy, 1993, 64), as the authors say they intended to do (Harman & Lorandos, 2021, p. 195). Effect coding evaluates the odds of an outcome occurring for a particular group compared to the population as a whole, rather than comparing all effects to a particular reference group (the standard approach). When using effect coding, the interpretation of the '1' value, in this case "fathers," must be compared to the average value for the overall sample, here represented by zero, *not* to the reference group coded as −1, in this case "mothers" (Hardy, 1993, 64). In testing the relationship of religious identity to political beliefs, a researcher may choose to code Catholics as −1, Lutherans as 1, Jews as 2, and Methodists as 3 to compare the beliefs of each group to the average beliefs across the entire population (represented as '0'), rather than only comparing Lutherans, Jews, and Methodists to a reference population of Catholics.

Harman and Lorandos' switch to the effect-coded approach means that when they attempt to interpret the coefficient of the "gender" term, they are interpreting the odds of something happening for fathers compared to average odds of that event happening overall (for fathers and mothers). Though they claim to be comparing fathers to mothers, saying, for example, "fathers had 1.73 greater odds … of losing custody of their child(ren) than did mothers" (197), this interpretation relies on the reported odds ratio that compares the value of '1' (fathers) to '0' (sample mean of mixed population), not '1' (fathers) to '-1' (mothers) (Jaquard and Turrisi, 24).

This error provides an independent reason that their conclusion about the relative odds of custody loss for father compared to mothers is incorrect, apart from the previously described errors. In Harman and Lorandos' coding approach, fathers are significantly more likely to lose custody than mothers, OR 1.73, $p = 0.002$ (Harman & Lorandos, 2021, p. 198, Table 5), but when we replicate the analysis using the coding detailed in the analytic plan (Table 4 above), this effect is not significant: OR 2.07, $p = 0.119$.

Harman and Lorandos' oft-repeated conclusion that fathers accused of alienation lose custody more often than mothers is an artifact of multiple statistical and coding errors. They fail to account for the presence of an interaction term when interpreting their regression output; they exclude 80% of cases from the custody loss analysis, injecting systematic bias; and they misinterpret their regression output due to deviations from the variable construction in their analytic plan. They report analyses from data they know contain significant mis-codings, which happen to be systematically biased by gender, while failing to report the corrected (and not statistically significant) results. These compounded errors mean their reported conclusions are not supported by their underlying data, *even if their dataset were appropriate.*

Re-analysis of part of Hypothesis 1 with corrected coding and regression methodology

Given that we are providing a commentary and not a replication study, we do not re-assess all of Harman and Lorandos' regression analyses here. We provide a re-analysis of the custody loss component of their Hypothesis 1, with the errors corrected (Meier et al., 2021).

In Table 5, we show the regression analysis correcting the data set to include all "no custody loss" cases, rather than just "custody gain" cases, and using Harman and Lorandos' analytic plan's standard coding of 0/1 for gender and alienation crediting. Rather than report the odds ratios and coefficients for the independent variables, which, as we described previously, cannot be properly interpreted on their own due to the presence of the interaction term, we present the predicted average marginal effects and their significance. The corrected findings indicate that, regardless of gender, "founded" alienation increases the frequency of custody loss by 14.07% as compared to *alleged* alienation, a statistically significant increase. This finding that custody loss is driven by founded alienation, not gender, is consistent with, not the opposite of, Meier et al.'s finding that "[b]oth mothers and fathers lose custody at identical rates when the court deems them an alienator" (Meier, 2020, p. 100; Meier et al., 2019, p.19). Contrary to Harman and Lorandos' claim, the corrected analysis shows that there is no significant gender difference in custody losses in response to an alienation claim: the predicted 3.11% difference between mothers' and fathers' custody losses is not statistically significant ($p = 0.194$). We show our analysis only for Hypothesis 1, but it demonstrates that Harman and Lorandos' key conclusions that mothers fare better than fathers in court, and that their study contradicts Meier et al.'s findings, are unsupported when the errors enumerated above are corrected.

Conclusion

We have argued that Harman and Lorandos' study constitutes neither a "direct and thorough test" of Meier et al.'s research, nor a credible analysis of the issues both studies seek to address. The statistical and non-statistical problems we have detailed are easily overlooked by those who are not steeped in social science research methodology or who are lulled by Harman and Lorandos' confident tone and presentation, replete with complex (if erroneous) claims about both their data and their analyses. Our labor-intensive deconstruction of their sampling method, coding, and analyses and interpretations of both their own and our results reveals fundamental problems at every stage.

We conclude by noting that the state of the discourse around these matters of critical importance to our courts and the well-being of children (and parents) is regrettable. There are genuinely important questions here – most fundamentally, how often are abuse allegations true, false, or knowingly fabricated in family court? How often are parental alienation claims deployed to nullify credible risk? Neither study can directly answer these questions, but they are at the root of the divide between those who espouse the view that parental alienation and false abuse allegations are common, and those who assert that abuse allegations are rarely fabricated but alienation is widely misused to deny credible abuse. Answering these questions requires reasoned and deliberate research and consideration by objective scholars and practitioners acting in good faith.

As is detailed our other article rebutting their critique (Meier et al., 2022, J. Fam. Ther., Child Dev., & Child Cust.), we believe the FCO study's empirically clean, careful accounting of court findings and decisions in these cases invites and compels this conversation. Rather than engage directly with our study's findings and implications, we fear that Harman and Lorandos' article is agenda-driven, filled with error, and does more to obfuscate the issues than to shed light on courts' practices.

Disclosure statement

No potential conflict of interest was reported by the authors.

Funding

The co-authors of this paper were partially funded by U.S. National Institute of Justice Award No.: NIJ-2014-MU-CX-0859 in producing the final summary overview referenced herein.

References

Araji, S. K., & Bosek, R. L. (2010). Domestic violence, contested child custody, and the courts: Findings from five studies. In M. T. Hannah & B. Goldstein (Eds.), *Domestic violence, abuse, and child custody: Legal strategies and policy issues* (pp. 6–2–6-7). Civic Research Institute, Inc.

Ai, C., & Norton, E. C. (2003). Interaction terms in logit and probit models, *Economics Letters*, *80*(1), 123–129.

Bemiller, M. (2008). When battered mothers lose custody: A qualitative study of abuse at home and in the court. *Journal of Child Custody*, *5*(3–4), 228–255. https://doi.org/10.1080/15379410802583742

Berg, R. (2011). Parental alienation analysis, domestic violence, and gender bias in Minnesota Courts. *Law & Inequality*, *29*(1), 5–31.

California Protective Parents Association. (2018). Research. Protective Mothers, Endangered Children. Retrieved July 8, 2021, from https://www.caprotectiveparents.org/research.

Council of California. (2021). What appellate justices do. Retrieved on December, 12, 2021, from https://www.courts.ca.gov/2827.htm.

Darlington, R. B., & Hayes, R. F. (2017). *Regression Analysis and Linear Models Concepts, Applications, and Implementation* (Guilford Press).

Harman, J. J., & Lorandos, D. (2021). Allegations of family violence in court: How parental alienation affects judicial outcomes. *Psychology, Public Policy and Law*, *27*(2), 187–208.

Harman, J., & Lorandos, D. (2020). *Parental Alienation Allegations in Family Court*, https://OSF.io/j9bh5/ ("Harman & Lorandos OSF")

Jaffe, P. G., Crooks, C. V., & Poisson, S. E. (2003). Common misconceptions in addressing domestic violence in child custody disputes. *Juvenile and Family Court Journal*, *54*(4), 57–67. https://doi.org/10.1111/j.1755-6988.2003.tb00086.x

Jaccard, J., & Turrisi, R. (2003). *Interaction Effects in Multiple Regression. (Little Green)*. https://doi.org/10.4135/9781412984522

Karaca-Mandic, P., Norton, E. D., & Dowd, B. (2012). Interaction terms in nonlinear models. *Health Services Research 47*(1), 255–274. https://doi.org/10.1111/j.1475-6773.2011.01314.x

Kornblum, L. S., & Pollack, D. (2018). Child abuse: Beware the 'unsubstantiated finding'. *Wisconsin Lawyer*, *91*, 8.

Meier, J. (2020). U.S. child custody outcomes in cases involving parental alienation and abuse allegations. *Journal of Social Welfare and Family Law*, *42*(1), 92–105. https://doi.org/10.1080/09649069.2020.1701941

Meier, J., & Dickson, S. (2017). Mapping gender: Shedding empirical light on family courts' treatment of cases involving abuse and alienation. *Journal of Child Custody, Law and Inequality 35*(2), 311–33.

Meier, J. (2019). User guide, child custody outcomes in cases involving parental alienation and abuse allegations, United States, 2005–2014. https://www.icpsr.umich.edu/web/NACJD/studies/37331/versions/V2/datasets

Meier, J., Dickson, S., Rosen, R., & O'Sullivan, C. (2021). *Analysis of* Harman & Lorandos 2020 *Data*, https://osf.io/qaeum/ ("Meier et al., OSF")

Meier, J., Dickson, S., Rosen, R., & O'Sullivan, C. (2022). The Trouble with Harman and Lorandos' *Parental Alienation Allegations in Family Court Study* (2020). *Journal of Family Trauma, Child Custody & Child Development*, *19*(3/4), 295-317. https://doi.org/10.1080/26904586.2022.2036286.

Meier, J., Dickson, S., Rosen, R., O'Sullivan, C., & Hayes, J. (2019). Child custody outcomes in cases involving parental alienation and abuse allegations, Final Report to National Institute of Justice, https://papers.ssrn.com/sol3/papers.cfm?abstract_id=3448062

Meier, J., Dickson, S., Rosen, R., O'Sullivan, C., & Hayes, J. (2014). Child custody outcomes in cases involving parental alienation and abuse allegations, Submitted proposal: April 25, 2014, NIJ-2014-3749, http://www.ncdsv.org/GWU_Child-Custody-Outcomes-in-Cases-Involving-Parental-Alientation-and-Abuse-Allegations_4-25-2014.pdf

One Mom's Battle. (2021). Formal complaint to UN denouncing the United States of America. Retrieved December 12, 2021, from https://www.onemomsbattle.com/blog/c3nxqpqj764qurf1ntculgirig09o5.

Silberg, J., Dallam, S., & Samson, E. (2013). Crisis in Family Court: Lessons from Turned-Around Cases, Final Report submitted to the Office on Violence against Women, Department of Justice, Award #2011-TA-AX-K006.

Silberg, J., & Dallam, S. (2019). Abusers gaining custody in family courts: A case series of overturned decisions. *Journal of Child Custody*, *16*(2), 140–169. https://doi.org/10.1080/15379418.2019.1613204

Smith, R., & Coukos, P. (1997). Fairness and accuracy in evaluations of domestic violence and child abuse in custody determinations. *Judges Journal*, *36*, 38.

Stark, D. P., Choplin, J. M., & Wellard, S. E. (2019). Properly accounting for domestic violence in child custody cases: An evidence-based analysis and reform proposal. *Michigan Journal of Gender & Law*, *26*(1), 1–119.

The Court Said: the Campaign for Survivor Family Justice. (2021). We will End the Inhumane Treatment and Suffering of Children in the Family Courts. Retrieved December 12, 2021, from https://www.thecourtsaid.org.

Attachment issues and reunification of parents and children

Jean Mercer

ABSTRACT

Attachment concepts offer guidance for parenting plans and reunification efforts for infants and young children, but because attachment behavior and motivation change with age, they are much less helpful for school age children and adolescents. Misunderstandings about attachment can lead to mistaken decisions. This paper presents information about attachment issues at different developmental stages and the ways attachment concepts and observations can be appropriately applied. Three reunification models are discussed in terms of attachment and other factors. One of the models is novel and is used to propose services that may facilitate reunification.

Attachment to and separation from parents are obvious themes when changes are made in child custody. Attachment concepts are fruitful sources of guidance for custody, parenting, and reunification decisions involving very young children, but are less helpful for older children and adolescents. When misapplied, however, attachment concepts can lead to wrong decisions for both young and older children. Unfortunately, there has been a tendency for courts to confuse attachment phenomena in young children with typical needs and behaviors of older children, and this needs to be corrected with accurate information. This paper will address research-based information about attachment and will discuss how attachment concepts can be useful in discussions of parenting plans and reunification problems.

Basic ideas of attachment

The term *attachment* refers to the tendency of human beings to show more positive attitudes and emotional reactions to familiar people than to strangers, especially under threatening or uncomfortable circumstances. This tendency is very strong in infants and young children, who clearly seek proximity to familiar attachment figures, but becomes more complex and less obvious with development through the lifespan. All primates show attachment behaviors toward familiar individuals under some circumstances, and it is thought that this tendency is an innate one that developed under evolutionary pressure.

Attachment behavior is not present in the first months of life, but emerges somewhere between 6 and 12 months in most cases, at about the same time that fear is first displayed by infants. Older infants and toddlers are fearful when approached by strangers and look to or move toward familiar persons, often crying if they cannot reach a familiar caregiver. They respond to separation from familiar persons with distress, and to abrupt, long-term separation with depression, apathy, and disturbances of eating and sleeping. The peak of distress about separation from attachment figures occurs between one and two years, and distress decreases as language ability and other cognitive skills improves. Nevertheless, preschoolers and even younger school age children may still show great distress over separation if they are sick, tired, or frightened.

Early attachment events are focused on familiar adult caregivers, who are strongly differentiated from strangers. However, the intense attachment of the young child gradually becomes the foundation for ways of thinking and feeling about social relations in general. These developing responses to other people are called an internal working model (IWM) of social relationships. The IWM is related to early attachment experiences but is also shaped and re-shaped by social interactions, both observed and experienced. As the IWM develops, responses to separation become less intense, and fear of strangers diminishes greatly except when they appear threatening. By middle childhood, children can generally handle both short and longer-term separations (for instance, school attendance and sleepaway camp) from familiar adults or contact with strangers with considerable ease, and are becoming more concerned with peer relationships than with family relationships, although family affection and care are still valued. In adolescence, peer relationships also include romantic and sexual connections which in many circumstances take precedence over adult caregivers. In adulthood, social, sexual, and parental behaviors are all associated with the IWM.

Attachment theory and its foundations

Like other theories, attachment theory is a framework that brings together a range of relevant concepts and empirical work. Also like other theories, attachment theory has gone through a number of changes since its inception (Mercer, 2006), and some of the original ideas have been replaced by others (see Bowlby, 1958; Rutter, 1995; 2002). For example, the initial form of attachment theory held that young children formed attachments to a single caregiver only (monotropy), but the current view is that multiple attachments are common.

Basic attachment theory

The basic idea of attachment theory is that young human beings are born without attachment but develop attachment behavior and emotions during the second half of the first year, as a result of social interactions with sensitive, responsive caregivers. Attachment is not an innate reaction to biologically-related individuals, not does it occur as a result of feeding or other care. However, attachment is a very robust developmental phenomenon and occurs in the great majority of young children, even when adult caregiving is not ideal.

Foundations of attachment theory in observable events

It would be neither ethical nor practical to use experimental methods to study attachment in young human beings. As a result, the foundations of attachment theory are in naturalistic observation or in "natural experiments" that compare groups of people who have had different experiences with caregivers in early life.

Systematic observations by Bowlby and by Robertson (see Van der Horst & van der Veer, 2009), on children isolated from their parents when hospitalized, showed that children do not experience fear of strangers and do not seek physical proximity to familiar people in the first few months of life. A child's attachment to caregivers begins between 6 and 12 months of age, and is most intense between about one and two years of age. In similar studies, it has been shown that toddlers become distressed when they are abruptly separated from familiar caregivers. Prolonged separation from caregivers causes distress in the toddlers, leads to apathy and temporary developmental regression, and is then followed by recovery over a period of months. As children grow older, however, they become increasingly tolerant of separation from familiar people, and although they may experience some distress, they are usually able to respond to the whole situation and not just to the loss of contact with a caregiver. Adolescents are usually able to cope well with weeks or months of separation and may choose to separate themselves from unhealthy relationships as well as showing a normative tendency to choose increasing separation from caregivers with whom they were previously intensely involved.

Longitudinal research

An essential question about attachment is: "To what extent can childhood attachment predict adult characteristics?" Because there are a multitude of variables that shape development, this question is best answered by longitudinal research in which a group of children is observed from infancy to adulthood, with measurement of attachment and other individual characteristics at intervals. This difficult and time-consuming research has been carried out in a 30-year study that concluded that no childhood attachment situation was of necessity associated with any specific adult outcome (Sroufe, 2005). This study suggests that just as anatomy is not destiny, childhood attachment is not destiny, but both anatomy and attachment seem to be factors that play some role in determining development.

Measures of attachment

Because attachment behavior and attitudes toward social relationships change with development, no single measure of attachment can be used for all. This aspect of attachment is essential, and misunderstandings about it can lead to mistaken decisions.

In the description of measures that follows, there will be no discussion of "bonding" or of "bonding studies". The term bonding applies to adult and not to child attitudes and behaviors (Erhart et al., 2020; Klaus et al., 1972). Bonding is most observable in parents whose children are from birth to a few months old, and it involves adult engrossment with the baby and preoccupation like "falling in love". There is no established protocol for measuring bonding.

Toddlers

Older infants and toddlers display obvious behaviors that are thought to indicate attachment. These include avoidance of strangers and seeking of proximity to a familiar person at times of discomfort or experienced threat. Toddlers can also be seen to use a familiar person as a secure base for exploration; they will explore a strange place when they can intermittently look to or return to a familiar person, but will not explore if there is no familiar person present.

Young children's attachment behaviors can be evaluated with a standardized method called the Strange Situation Paradigm (Ainsworth et al., 1978). In this protocol, which was developed entirely for research and not for clinical purposes, a toddler and a familiar caregiver come into a prepared room where there are toys. The caregiver leaves briefly and then returns. (Many details are omitted here). The focus is on the child's behavior at the time of reunion with the caregiver.

Child reunion behavior was initially classified into three categories (Ainsworth et al., 1978), but a fourth category was later added (Main & Solomon, 1986). These categories are based on behavior toward the caregiver: is the child easily comforted by the caregiver? Does the child "snub" the caregiver to begin with? Is the child distressed, angry, and difficult to comfort? Does the child behave in strongly atypical ways?

Toddlers who are easily soothed on reunion with the caregiver are said to be securely attached, and typically this is characteristic of about 65% of young children. The approximately 20% who actively avoid and "snub" the returning caregiver but later accept the caregiver are said to be insecure-avoidant. Another 15% are placed in the insecure-ambivalent category; they seek the caregiver but also resist the caregiver and are hard to "settle" (Teti & Nakagawa, 1990). A small number of toddlers fall into a disorganized/disoriented attachment category; they seem dazed or fearful when the caregiver returns and may back toward the caregiver or fall to the floor (Main & Solomon, 1986).

The categories used are descriptive of the quality of attachment behavior. There is no measure of "strength" of attachment. In addition, the categories are descriptive of behavior within a given relationship and are not necessarily indicative of how a young child would behave with a different caregiver.

Preschoolers and kindergarteners

The attachment behavior that is so evident in toddlers becomes less common as children age and, as a result, is more difficult to classify. There are assessment methods for preschoolers (Cassidy et al., 1992) and for 6-year-olds (Crittenden, 2006).

School-age children and adolescents

Children of school age still prefer familiar caregivers under distressing circumstances, but their attachment behavior is hard to evaluate, and they are not yet able to talk about attachment issues as adults can. Adolescents, however, may be able to respond to the Adult Attachment Interview, a series of interview questions for which responses can be scored as indicating that the respondent is currently autonomous (secure) about social relationships, dismissing, preoccupied, or disorganized (Bakermans-Kranenburg & van Ijzendoorn, 2009).

Uses and abuses of the attachment concept in legal decisions

An accurate understanding of attachment can help lead to decisions about child custody and parenting that are beneficial to children's development. Misunderstandings can cause decisions that are potentially harmful to children. Two points are essential to good use of attachment concepts. First, how attachment functions is largely dependent on age and developmental stage. Second, attachment is not the only factor that makes for good development, and overuse of attachment concepts carries the potential for harmful decisions in courts and in other governmental and administrative areas (see Woolgar & Scott, 2014).

Making decisions about individuals: Creating and modifying parenting plans

Attachment considerations are most important for parenting plans involving infants and young children. Although children from birth to 6 months have not yet developed attachment, plans should be made to give them frequent experiences with any caregiver they will later be expected to have contact with. The young infant's apparent nonchalance about changes of caregiver is not permanent, and there will eventually be strong protests against the approach of adults, including infrequently-seen parents, who are classed by the infant as "strangers" because of unfamiliarity. These developmentally typical changes are easily misinterpreted by parents (and by the court) as evidence that someone has mistreated the child and/or caused fear of the less familiar parent.

If attachment has occurred to one parent and not the other, older infants and toddlers can be expected to protest vigorously against separation from one parent and the approach of the other. This is distressing to parents, but is completely expectable and should be planned for. Young children adapt to separations over time (Field, 1991), but there is less emotional distress for everyone if changes in contact are made gradually. Interacting with an unfamiliar person in a familiar place is less distressing for infants than being in a strange place with a strange person. Short periods of contact will become less and less distressing and then can be lengthened and the venue changed. Although caregivers want to feed the child, it is not likely that an upset child will take any food, so this should wait. The issue is not just to save the child unnecessary distress, but to prevent the unfamiliar caregiver from negative emotions that may cause giving up contact, anger at the familiar caregiver, or both. In cases where visitation is supervised, it is important that the supervisor understands these issues and also knows that interactions under supervision are not necessarily what would occur otherwise.

Attempts have been made to argue that overnight visitation with young children should be delayed to age 4 years (McIntosh et al., 2014). Evidence supporting this viewpoint was very weak and was critiqued effectively by Warshak (2018). Overnight stays are potentially distressing to young children, as they are longer than most daytime visits and children often depend on familiar bedtime rituals that may not be known to less familiar caregivers. Co-sleeping with a parent may be an issue, particularly as it may be interpreted by adults as having a sexual aspect. However, calm overnight stays can be worked toward by gradual steps, as long as parents and courts are aware that young children can show distress and need to be comforted in these situations. It is helpful to the child if "transitional objects" (Winnicott, 1993) like blankets, stuffed animals, and pacifiers are available when the child is with the less familiar parent.

From age 3 or 4, as the child's language and concepts of time improve, visiting becomes easier and more gratifying. However, changes in lengths of visits still need to be gradual if possible. Going from a single overnight to a week-long visit is likely to be uncomfortable. However, using phone calls, Zoom, and so on to allow regular contact with the more familiar parent can be of great help.

From school age on, children become accustomed to separation and may choose it (overnight with a friend, sleepaway camp). Their attachment needs and behavior are typically reduced by this time and parenting plans can be based on other factors. The fact that school children need to be warned not to go with strangers is evidence that their social relationships have developed considerably since the early time when attachment to familiar caregivers was a paramount motivation.

Making decisions about individuals: Failing to consider developmental change

A review of child custody decisions in one state's courts showed that judges had made decisions based on a range of misunderstandings about attachment (Mercer, 2006). One judge opined that a 12-month-old was too young to have formed an attachment to a caregiver, whereas in fact a child of that age typically shows intense attachment behavior, distress on separation, and strong avoidance of unfamiliar people. In another case, the judge stated that a 16-year-old would have severe emotional damage as a result of separation from a familiar caregiver. In fact, although there might be many reasons why a change of custody for a teenager might be harmful, a break in attachment is not one of them, as teenagers are already engaged in strengthening social relationships with their peers and others outside the family.

Attachment concepts can be helpful in custody decisions for older infants and toddlers from about 6 months to 2–3 years of age. They are not helpful for infants from birth to about 6 months of age, as these young infants have not yet developed fearful responses to strange people or events and are not distressed at a change of caregiver (provided that they are well cared for). During the preschool period and afterward, children become more and more capable of adapting to changing caregivers, as we see in their relationships with teachers and others outside the family, although they may continue to prefer one caregiver over another for a variety of reasons.

Individual decisions and measures of attachment

The attachment measures discussed earlier in this paper were never intended to make individual legal or clinical decisions. They were developed for research purposes and used to compare groups, not individuals. There have been efforts to use the Strange Situation Paradigm to recommend custody for one parent and not the other (George et al., 2011), but such use is contrary to the purpose of the method. Attachment measures unfortunately do not offer a simple method of making custody decisions.

Attachment measures and insecurity

Attachment measures for children allow classification of a child's attachment to a caregiver into several categories. Two of these describe the child's attachment as "insecure". It is important to realize that the "insecure" categories are part of the normal range of attachment, as is the "secure" category. About 30% of children are classified as having a form of "insecure" attachment, and this is not an attachment disorder (Teti & Nakagawa, 1990).

Toddlers and preschoolers who are devoted to transitional objects (Winnicott, 1993) like "security blankets" or stuffed toys should not be regarded as "insecure" on this account, and the use of a transitional object should not be attributed to ill-treatment or to attachment problems. In cases where there is abrupt custody change or visitation is going badly, toddlers and preschoolers need to be helped to have transitional objects with them. The same is true for pacifiers or thumb-sucking, even when a child might be regarded as "too old" for these practices. Custody and parenting plans should not be altered on the basis of young children's behaviors of this kind.

Disorganized/disoriented attachment

The idea of disorganized attachment (Main & Hesse, 1990) was mentioned earlier in this paper. It is concerning when children display unusual behavior on reunion with a caregiver, but it is important to remember that they may show much more typical behavior with other familiar people. It is thought that caregivers who trigger disorganized attachment behavior do so as a result of their own unresolved trauma. They look frightened when they see the child, and the child, responding with fear to an adult's fearful face, tries to approach while not looking at the fearful expression. The appropriate treatment for this situation is directed at helping the traumatized caregiver, not removing the child from contact with this familiar person. It is certainly wrong to assume that disorganized attachment is proof of maltreatment.

Granqvist et al. (2017) called attention to the increased interest in disorganized attachment in recent years. They noted that the interest was in part dependent on false assumptions that "attachment measures can be used as definitive assessments of the individual in forensic/child protection settings... that disorganized attachment... reliably indicates child maltreatment, ...is a strong predictor of pathology, and... represents a fixed or static 'trait' of the child, impervious to development or help" (p. 534).

Attachment disorders

There are two attachment disorders listed in DSM-5 (American Psychiatric Association, 2013), and both of them are likely to be related to previous institutionalization, foster care, or adoption. One of these disorders is Reactive Attachment Disorder, a psychiatric disorder of young children characterized by social withdrawal, sadness, and apathy, following a period of many separations or by disengaged care by many caregivers, typical of institutional care. Allen & Schuengel (2020) have discussed how the actual characteristics of this disorder differ from those popularly conceived as identifying it). The second attachment disorder, Disinhibited Social Engagement Disorder, is related to the same kind of background experiences but is notable for the ready engagement of the child with strangers and the lack of separation anxiety, very different from what is seen in the typically-developing child of this age. Children with either of these conditions need special handling and it would not be advisable to subject them to changes of custody or of parenting plans unless there are serious reasons for doing so. Children with DSED may easily be thought to be independent, friendly, and gregarious, characteristics that are valued and approved in the Western world, but it would be a mistake to think that their apparently easy transitions from one to another caregiver are evidence that transitions are in their best interest. Many changes of caregiver, with the demands they place on the child to adapt repeatedly to new places, people, rules, and ways of communicating, are likely to interfere with children's development of desirable preschool social and emotional skills like cognitive and emotional empathy. In addition, at a more immediate level, incautious children may be easily lured or groomed by predatory adults.

Attachment and models of reunification

Estrangement of parents and children may result from a wide range of causes, including simple loss of contact over a period of time. Children may actively resist contact because they respond to a parent as if he or she were a stranger ("estrangement"), because there have been accidental negative experiences with the parent, because the parent has poor parenting skills, because there have been experiences of domestic violence, because the parent has been abusive, or because a preferred parent has encouraged the child's refusal (a situation referred to as "parental alienation"). Under any of these circumstances, a decision may be made to seek reunification of the child with the rejected parent. An important first step in this decision is to follow a protocol for ruling out causes of estrangement like previous abuse (see, for example, Milchman, 2021), but this is far from a universal practice.

The term "reunification" was initially used to refer to situations where a child who had been in foster care was returned to the custody of the biological family. In recent years, the term "reunification" in forensic settings has come to refer to forms of treatment used in cases where children of divorced couples reject contact with one parent. These children may be described as estranged, or, in cases where the preferred parent is thought to have encouraged the rejection, "alienated" from the rejected parent. Reunification efforts can follow several different models.

The attachment model

The possible association between reunification and attachment is an obvious one. In attachment, children develop a strong preference for and tendency to seek a familiar caregiver such as a parent. In estrangement, the child avoids a parent and prefers the other parent, suggesting that attachment to one parent, if it existed, has been damaged and needs to be restored. It is plausible that attachment concepts could provide a model for reunification when children are young.

The premise that estrangement or alienation results from damage to attachment has been brought up from time to time by practitioners focused on reunification of children and rejected divorced parents. Richard Gardner (2002), the originator of the parental alienation concept, referenced this in a 2002 book, apparently considering some outmoded tenets of attachment theory. One current practitioner bases his entire theory on the idea that a child's attachment to a parent has been "suppressed" if the child rejects that parent (Childress, 2015).

Whether attachment could or could not play a role in rejection of a parent, and therefore in reunification with the parent, is a matter that depends on the child's age. As shown throughout this paper, attachment and attachment behaviors are modified as an individual develops from birth to adulthood, with intense attachment behavior between about 6 months and 2–3 years, and rapid decreases in the ensuing years. The attachment behavior toward caregivers characteristic of the early years later modulates into a range of social relationships with both familiar and unfamiliar people. The role of attachment in relationships with parents also modulates.

Attachment measures versus age as factors in parenting plans

As was noted before in this paper, attachment measures like the Strange Situation Paradigm (Ainsworth et al., 1978) were intended to compare populations for research purposes, not to assess individuals for forensic or clinical purposes. Such measures are also time-consuming, and few practitioners are trained to use them, so they are not useful to courts. Fortunately, the age of a typically-developing child is an excellent proxy measurement that gives insight into attachment needs and probable responses to separations and reunions.

Atypical development

Children who are not developing typically may respond rather differently than other children their age to changes in parenting plans or custody. Children with autistic spectrum disorder (ASD) may be extremely distressed by changes, and this distress may affect their functioning for months. Children with cerebral palsy (CP) or other neurological disorders may also be particularly vulnerable, especially if the disorder affects their communication abilities. Children with emotional disorders like oppositional and defiant disorder (ODD) or attention disorders, depression, or anxiety disorders may need to be considered in terms of their particular mood and behavioral tendencies. Any type of intellectual or developmental delays may mean that a child needs to be thought of in terms of his or her actual developmental progress rather than chronological age.

Very young infants

As was noted earlier in this paper, infants between birth and 6 months have not developed attachment behavior or the associated fear reactions to strange people or events. Visiting or custody changes do not need to consider current attachment issues, although it would be wise during this period to plan ahead to the time when a child will be concerned about separations and strangers.

Visitation and periods of care by each parent can begin shortly after birth. The only caveat here is that if breastfeeding is planned, it would be wise to postpone any other sort of feeding for at least two weeks, until lactation is established. Breastfeeding is not known to be associated with attachment and should not be thought of as a way in which a child's mother will somehow gain attachment superiority over the father.

Infants in the early months are accepting and responsive in a developmentally-appropriate way to any smiling, playful person, strange or familiar, and 4–5-month-olds are particularly friendly and sociable. If an infant of this age shows discomfort or distress with a particular adult, there may be a number of reasons unrelated to attachment for this. These could range from clumsiness and poor parenting skills, to unfamiliarity with the child's eating and sleeping habits, to experiences of abuse associated with the parent. The reasons should be explored if infant distress is observed, but it may well be that the parent needs support and guidance in infant care and there has been no abuse.

Older infants and toddlers

At some point between 6 and 12 months of age, children typically begin to react with fear to unfamiliar people and events. When frightened or distressed, they try to stay near familiar caregivers. At this stage, and on until the age of 2 years or more, children respond to an unfamiliar biological parent as they would to any other stranger and are upset if left alone with that person. Unless there is actual evidence of abuse, or if an older toddler discloses abuse, it should never be assumed that the child's behavior indicates past or present abuse by anyone.

Parents who are trying to reunify with a toddler whom they have not seen for some time need to be made aware of these facts and helped to work toward an attachment relationship gradually. This can be painful for a rejected parent, as it requires interaction with the other parent and maintenance of a playful "courtship" of the child that may be a completely unfamiliar way for an adult to behave. It is easy for a parent to abandon the effort and leave the child's life temporarily or permanently, or alternatively to blame the other parent for the child's attitude.

Infants and toddlers who have visited a less familiar parent often both cling to and act angry toward the more familiar parent on return. This is, again, typical attachment behavior for this age and should not in itself be taken as evidence of abuse.

Parenting plans for children at this stage need to recognize attachment and separation issues and to encourage parents to invest time and patience in order to create attachment relationships on which continuing more mature relationships can be founded.

Preschool children

Typically-developing children from about age 3 years on still have some concerns about separation from familiar people, but their capacity to understand and use language helps them tolerate situations that would have caused great distress in earlier months. However, preschoolers are still easily frightened by rough, noisy, or abrupt adult behavior that may have been attended as joking or play. Many preschoolers are afraid of masks or costumes and dislike clowns or other people who behave "peculiarly". Parents who are attempting to reunify with a preschooler whom they have not seen for a while need to be aware of these forms of fearfulness.

Reunification with a preschooler is much less influenced by attachment issues, but in addition to considering child fears, parents should be aware that telling the child what will happen and using preschool time concepts ("when we wake up" rather than tomorrow) can make the process more comfortable for everyone.

School age children

Children of 6 years or older still prefer to be with familiar caregivers when they are sick or frightened, but cam enjoy time with less familiar people and use that time to develop more mature relationships with them. They may still miss the familiar home and more familiar caregiver, but can be helped on this by phone or Zoom contacts. When away from the familiar home, they may wish most for play and contacts with other children their age.

Adolescents

Typically-developing adolescents have relationships with adults that are far more mature than the toddler's attachment relations. They may miss or be concerned about a familiar parent when away, but they are more likely to long for contact with peers, both friends and possible romantic partners. By this point in development, attachment issues are a negligible aspect of reunification, which is far more likely to be influenced by past family history and present parent attitudes and conduct.

The parental alienation model

In some cases, estrangement of a child from a parent may be rightly or wrongly attributed to a preferred parent's encouragement of the child's rejection of the other parent. This situation has been called parental alienation (Gardner, 1985; Warshak, 2010), a term that is sometimes applied to the child's estrangement and sometimes to whatever the preferred parent has done to encourage or cause the estrangement.

"Reunification therapies", in the parental alienation context, are methods that purport to reduce the estrangement and create an improved relationship between the child and the rejected parent. These include Family Bridges (Warshak, 2010, 2019), High Road to Reunification (Conscious Co-Parenting Institute, n.d.), Turning Points (Gottlieb, 2012), Overcoming Barriers (Sullivan et al., 2010), and Transitioning Families (also used for reunification after nonfamilial abduction; Judge et al., 2016). Reunification therapies are usually done at court order and include a period of prohibited contact with the preferred parent. Interestingly, advocates of these treatments generally speak of them as "psychoeducation" and deny that they are psychotherapies. Nevertheless, it is common to refer to practitioners as reunification therapists, rather than educators.

Although reunification may be desired in a variety of circumstances, reunification therapies are used entirely in cases where parental alienation is alleged to be the cause of the estrangement. Other causes of estrangement, like a period without contact or experiences of abuse, are not the focus of these treatments. Reunification therapies like Family Bridges appear to be used primarily with children from about 9–17 years of age, although younger children have been the subjects of parental alienation allegations. It remains unclear how children are identified as candidates for these therapies, as there seems to be no established protocol for deciding that parental alienation is present

Critiques of outcome research on reunification therapies have concluded that only weak evidence of their effectiveness has been published (Mercer, 2019a, 2019b). Although parental alienation advocates often put forward the argument that children need both parents, reports of treatment outcomes generally consider only the satisfaction of the previously-rejected parent as a criterion and fail to note whether the child has adequate relationships with both parents after the treatment. Court-ordered prohibitions of contact with the preferred parent may be renewed for years.

A family preservation/reunification model

The principle of family preservation and reunification states that there is benefit in maintaining connections between parents and children in circumstances where they may be or have been separated (Lloyd, 2020). This concept originated in consideration of children who had been placed in foster care because of family problems (including abuse) and who now might be reunited with the biological family.

Reunification of children with estranged parents is not identical with reunification of foster children with their biological parents, but the analogy is clear, with the major difference that children of divorce have usually remained living with one parent, while foster children have been separated from both parents and have lived with foster parents to whom they may have become attached or accustomed. In both cases, a child is asked to transition from one familiar type of social setting to another which is unfamiliar and about which he or she may feel quite ambivalent, if not wholly opposed.

Reunification services for families whose children have been in foster care often include substance abuse and domestic violence services, as these problems are common factors in foster placement of children. These problems need to be corrected before reunification is attempted. Such problems may or may not contribute to a child's estrangement from a divorced parent, but if they have been present but are now corrected, provision of services may help to reconcile the child to contact with the parent.

Mental health services

Reunification of children with parents under any circumstances is more likely to be effective if mental health problems are treated effectively before the reunification attempt. Children's reluctance to have contact with a parent may be related to anxiety disorders, issues connected with autism, or similar problems. Children who are physically or mentally disabled may also need mental health support. One or both parents may also bring anxiety, depression, problems with anger management, and so on, into the reunification attempt, if these have not been controlled earlier.

Help with parenting skills and relationships

In family preservation/reunification situations, which may be analogous to reunification with a divorced parent, the provision of help to the parents may increase the probability of successful reunification by improving parenting skills and parent-child relationships.

During the infant-toddler period, when attachment is a serious issue for reunification, parents can benefit from attachment-related treatments. Circle of Security (Woodhouse et al., 2018) is a program directed to informing parents about attachment processes and behavior and thus supporting children's attachment. Circle of Security has considerable research support but is not an evidence-based treatment (Mercer, 2015). Attachment and Biobehavioral Catch-up (ABC; Dozier & Bernard, 2019) is an evidence-based program that focuses on sensitizing foster parents to the subtle attachment communications shown by young children in care. Either of these programs could be useful for divorced parents whose young children avoid or reject them.

A number of programs that address parenting skills have been used to support family preservation/reunification efforts (Lloyd, 2020). By analogy, these may also be helpful in parent-child reunification following divorce. Some of the relevant programs that have strong research support are Incredible Years (Webster-Stratton et al., 2011), Parent-Child Interaction Therapy (PCIT; Hood & Eyberg, 2003), and Positive Parenting Program (Triple-P; Pickering & Sanders, 2015). However, as Lloyd (2020) has pointed out, "Despite the evidence that these programs cause positive changes in parent-child interactions, parenting skills, and child behavior, research investigating whether... parent training programs increase likelihood of reunification is limited" (p. 1973) even with respect to family preservation/reunification efforts. There is no research on use of these programs following child rejection of a divorced parent, but the analogy between family preservation/reunification and reunification after divorce makes the programs worth considering. Programs supporting parenting skills have the advantages over parental alienation-model treatments that they are much less expensive and do not require a court order for separation of the child from the preferred parent.

Conclusion

The concept of attachment provides important guidance for parenting plans and custody decisions affecting infants and toddlers. It may thus assist in reunification of divorced parents with children who avoid or reject them. Attention to attachment issues can help facilitate reunification of young children with unfamiliar parents by helping children stay calm and engaged with the adults. Young children's attachment behaviors and related emotional responses can easily be misinterpreted to mean that they have experienced abuse from an unfamiliar person when this has never happened. When young children's attachment needs are ignored, their distress can also convince each parent that the other must have harmed or in some way manipulated the child, when this is not the case. Child distress and its misinterpretations can lead to avoidable problems with parenting plans and even trigger allegations of abuse and of parental alienation. Preschool children are less likely to show attachment-related concerns but may still do so if tired, hungry, sick, or frightened in unfamiliar situations.

Attachment issues are of much less importance for school age children than for the younger groups. Children of this age are involved in relationships with adults, including parents, teachers, stepparents, grandparents, older siblings, neighbors, and so on. These relationships are not in the true sense attachment relationships, as the older people are not generally needed to act as a secure bases and allow the children to explore and learn. To the extent that an adult has been a comforting, trustworthy caregiver, a child will experience distress on extended separation, will miss the adult, and will wish to reunite, but the distress will be much less severe and disabling than the distress felt by a separated younger child. School age children may choose separations in order to take part in desired activities. A school age child who rejects a parent does not do so because of attachment to the preferred parent or lack of attachment to the rejected parent, but has more complex reasons for the rejection.

Adolescents like to be able to choose contact with a loved parent but to do so on their own terms. Their social relationships now focus on peers and on romantic possibilities rather than on family. Rejection of a parent is not attachment-related, but occurs for a wide range of reasons, including the adolescent's need for autonomy.

Because of these developmental changes, an attachment model of reunification work is useful primarily for children under 3 years of age, though it may be extended to age 5 or 6. Reunification work focused on parental alienation is also limited in applicability. Its usefulness depends on accurate identification of parental alienation as a cause of estrangement and there appears to be no established protocol for doing this. Unfortunately, treatments intended for reunification of children in parental alienation cases have not been adequately supported by well-designed, well-implemented research. These treatments are most often used with older school age children and adolescents, for whom issues of attachment to parents are of little significance.

An analogy can be drawn between efforts to reunify a divorced parent with a rejecting child and efforts to reunify children who have been in foster care with their biological parents. Younger foster children and their parents may benefit from treatments aimed at improving the parents' knowledge of child attachment behavior and their responses to it. Evidence-based programs for improving parenting skills have been used with older foster children and adolescents as they return to their biological families, but it remains unclear whether those programs actually increase the likelihood of successful reunification. There is presently no research showing the effects of parenting skills programs on the outcomes of efforts to reunify parents with estranged children, but, given that attachment methods are age-limited and parental alienation methods are poorly supported by evidence, parenting skills improvement would seem to be a reasonable alternative in estrangement cases.

Disclosure of interest

The authors report no conflicts of interest. The authors alone are responsible for the content and writing of the paper.

Ethical standards and informed consent

No human subjects were involved in this study.

ORCID

Jean Mercer http://orcid.org/0000-0003-3217-3953

References

Ainsworth, M., Blehar, M., Waters, E., & Wall, S. (1978). *Patterns of attachment*. Erlbaum.

Allen, B., & Schuengel, C. (2020). Attachment disorders diagnosed by community practitioners: A replication and extension. *Child and Adolescent Mental Health*, *25*(1), 4–10. https://doi.org/10.1111/camh.12338

American Psychiatric Association. (2013). *Diagnostic and statistical manual of mental disorders*. Author.

Bakermans-Kranenburg, M., & van Ijzendoorn, M. (2009). The first 10,000 Adult Attachment Interviews: Distributions of adult attachment representations in clinical and non-clinical groups. *Attachment & Human Development*, *11*(3), 223–263. https://doi.org/10.1080/14616730902814762

Bowlby, J. (1958). The nature of a child's tie to his mother. *International Journal of Psychoanalysis*, *39*, 350–433.

Cassidy, J., & Marvin, R.; the MacArthur Attachment Working Group (1992). *Attachment organization in preschool children: Procedures and coding manual*. 4th ed.. Unpublished manuscript, University of Virginia.

Childress, C. (2015). *An attachment-based model of parental alienation: Foundations*. Oaksong Press.

Conscious Co-parenting Institute. (n.d.). *Overview of the high road to family reunification program*. Unpublished paper.

Crittenden, P. (2006). Why do inadequate parents do what they do? In O. Mayseless (Ed.), *Parenting representations* (pp. 388–434). Cambridge University Press. https://doi.org/10.1017/CBO9780511499869.014

Dozier, M., & Bernard, K. (2019). *Coaching parents of vulnerable infants: The attachment and biobehavioral catchup approach*. Guilford.

Erhart, A., Olsavsky, A., & Kim, P. (2020). Bonding. In S. Hupp & J. Jewell (Eds.), *Encyclopedia of child and adolescent development* (Vol. 6, pp. 1853–1866). Wiley. https://doi.org/10.1002/9781119171492.wecad201

Field, T. (1991). Young children's adaptations to repeated separations from their mothers. *Child Development*, *62*(3), 539–547. https://doi.org/10.1111/j.1467-8624.1991.tb01550.x

Gardner, R. (1985). Recent trends in divorce and custody litigation. *The Academy Forum*, *29* (2), 3–7.

Gardner, R. (2002). *Therapeutic interventions for children with parental alienation syndrome*. Creative Therapeutics.

George, C., Isaacs, M., & Marvin, R. (2011). Incorporating attachment assessments into custody evaluations: The case of a 2-year-old and her parents. *Journal of Child Custody*, *49*, 483–500. https://doi.org/10.1111/j.1744-1617.201.01386.x

Gottlieb, L. (2012). *The parental alienation syndrome: A family therapy and collaborative system approach to amelioration*. Charles C. Thomas.

Granqvist, P., Sroufe, L. A., Dozier, M., Hesse, E., Steele, M., van Ijzendoorn, M., Solomon, J., Schuengel, C., Fearon, P., Bakermans-Kranenburg, M., Steele, H., Cassidy, J., Carlson, E., Madigan, S., Jacobvitz, D., Foster, S., Behrens, K., Rifkin-Graboi, A., Gribneau, N., … Duschinsky, R. (2017). Disorganized attachment in infancy: A review of the phenomenon and its implications for clinicians and policy-makers. *Attachment & Human Development*, *19*(6), 534–558. https://doi.org/10.1080/14616734.2017.1354040

Hood, K., & Eyberg, S. (2003). Outcomes of parent-child interaction therapy: Mothers' reports of maintenance three to six years after treatment. *Journal of Clinical Child and Adolescent Psychology*, *32*(3), 419–430. https://doi.org/10.1207/S15374424JCCP3203_10

Judge, A., Bailey, R., Behrman-Lippert, J., Bailey, E., Psaila, C., & Dickel, J. (2016). The transitioning families therapeutic reunification model in nonfamilial abductions. *Family Court Review*, *54*(2), 232–249. https://doi.org/10.1111/fcre.12215

Klaus, M., Jerauld, R., Kreger, N., McAlpine, W., Steffa, M., & Kennell, J. (1972). Maternal attachment. *New England Journal of Medicine*, *286*(9), 460–463. https://doi.org/10.1056/NEJM197203022860904

Lloyd, M. (2020). Family preservation and reunification programs. In S. Hupp & J. Jewell (Eds.), *Encyclopedia of child and adolescent development* (Vol. 5, pp. 1967–1978. Wiley. https://doi.org/10.1002/9781119171492.wecad212

Main, M., & Hesse, E. (1990). Parents' unresolved traumatic experiences are related to infants' insecure-disorganized/disoriented attachment status: Is frightened or frightening behavior the linking mechanism? In M. Greenberg, D. Cicchetti, & M. Cummings (Eds.), *Attachment in the preschool years* (pp. 161–182). University of Chicago Press.

Main, M., & Solomon, J. (1986). Discovery of a new, insecure disorganized/disoriented attachment pattern. In M. Yogman & T.B. Brazelton (Eds.), *Affective development in infancy* (pp. 95–129). Ablex.

McIntosh, J., Pruett, M., & Kelly, J. (2014). Parental separation and overnight care of young children, Part II: Putting theory into practice. *Family Court Review*, *52*(2), 256–262. https://doi.org/10.1111/fcre.12088

Mercer, J. (2006). *Understanding attachment*. Praeger.

Mercer, J. (2015). Examining circle of security: A review of research and theory. *Research on Social Work Practice*, *25*(3), 382–392. https://doi.org/10.1177/1049731536620

Mercer, J. (2019a). Are parental alienation treatments safe and effective for children and adolescents?*Journal of Child Custody*, *16*(1), 67–111. https://doi.org/10.1080/15379418.2018.1557578

Mercer, J. (2019b). Examining parental alienation treatments: Problems with principles and practices. *Child and Adolescent Social Work Journal, 36*(4), 351–363. https://doi.org/10.1007/s10560-019-00625-8

Milchman, M. (2021). Assessing causes of children's parent rejection in child custody cases: Differentiating parental alienation from child sexual abuse, psychological maltreatment, and bad parenting. In R. Geffner, J. White, L. Hamberger, V. Vaughan-Eden, & V. Vieth (Eds.), *Handbook of interpersonal violence and abuse across the lifespan.* Springer Nature. https://doi.org/10.1007/978-3-319-62122-7_318-1

Pickering, J., & Sanders, M. (2015). The triple P-positive parenting program. *Family Matters, 96*, 53–63.

Rutter, M. (1995). Clinical implications of attachment concepts. Retrospect and prospect. *Journal of Child Psychology and Psychiatry, 36*, 599–571. https://doi.org/10.1111/j.1469-7610-1905.tb02314.x

Rutter, M. (2002). Nature, nurture, and development: From evangelism through science toward policy and practice. *Child Development, 73*(1), 1–21. https://doi.org/10.1111/1467-8624.00388

Sroufe, L. A. (2005). Attachment and development: A prospective, longitudinal study from birth to adulthood. *Attachment & Human Development, 7*(4), 349–367. https://doi.org/10.1080/14616730500365928

Sullivan, M., Ward, P., & Deutsch, R. (2010). Overcoming barriers family camp: A program for high-conflict divorced families when a child is resisting contact with a parent. *Family Court Review, 48*(1), 116–135. https://doi.org/10.1111/j.1744-1617.2009.01293.x

Teti, D., & Nakagawa, M. (1990). Assessing attachment in infancy: The strange situation and alternative systems. In E. Gibbs & D. Teti (Eds.), *Interdisciplinary assessment of infants* (pp. 191–214). P.H. Brookes.

Van der Horst, F., & van der Veer, R. (2009). Separation and divergence: The untold story of James Robertson's and John Bowlby's theoretical dispute on mother-child separation. *Journal of the History of the Behavioral Sciences, 45*(3), 236–252. https://doi.org/10.1002/jhbs.20380

Warshak, R. (2010). Family bridges: Using insights from social science to reconnect parents and alienated children. *Family Court Review, 48*(1), 48–80. https://doi.org/10.1111/j.1744-1617.2009.01288.x

Warshak, R. (2018). Night shifts: Revisiting blanket restrictions on children's overnights with separated parents. *Journal of Divorce & Remarriage, 59*(4), 282–323. https://doi.org/10.1080/10502556.2018.1454193

Warshak, R. (2019). Reclaiming parent-child relationships: Outcomes of family bridges with alienated children. *Journal of Divorce & Remarriage, 60*(8), 645–667. https://doi.org/10.1080/10502556.2018.1529505

Webster-Stratton, C., Rinaldi, J., & Reid, J. (2011). Long-term outcomes of incredible years parenting program: Predictors of adolescent adjustment. *Child and Adolescent Mental Health, 16*(1), 38–46. https://doi.org/10.1111/j.1475-3588.2010.00576.x

Winnicott, D. (1993). Transitional objects and transitional phenomena: A study of the first not-me possession. In G. Pollock (Ed.), *Pivotal papers on identification* (pp. 139–157). International Universities Press.

Woodhouse, S., Powell, B., Cooper, G., Hoffman, K., & Cassidy, J. (2018). The Circle of Security intervention: Design, research, and implementation. In H. Steele & M. Steele (Eds.), *Handbook of attachment-based interventions* (pp. 50–78). Guilford.

Woolgar, M., & Scott, S. (2014). The negative consequences of over-diagnosing attachment disorders in adopted children: The importance of comprehensive formulations. *Clinical Child Psychology and Psychiatry, 19*(3), 355–366. https://doi.org/10.1177/1359104513478545

Parental sobriety and parent-child reunification in dependency court: Does the 15-month Adoption and Safe Families Act (ASFA) rule support parent-child reunification?

Eileen M. Ahlin, Don Hummer and Mitra Honardoost

ABSTRACT

With the number of Americans suffering from addiction at an all-time high, child protective and social services agencies need a coordinated response to ensure that children spend less time in foster care. The Adoption and Safe Families Act (ASFA) of 1997 sought to improve the permanency process by specifying a timeline to parental reunification. The ASFA 15-month rule places limitations on the time frame in which a parent must achieve sobriety before parent-child reunification can occur. The present study assesses the impact of the ASFA 15-month rule on children's permanency outcomes among children placed in out-of-home care due to parental substance use. First, we examine whether there are differences in permanency outcomes across the various circumstances that lead to out-of-home placements. Next, we explore whether child characteristics influence parent-child reunification based on the reason for out-of-home placement. Results show that alternate permanency solutions to parental reunification are more likely for younger children and when multiple children are removed from the home. Implications for these findings are discussed, as are directions for future research.

Children raised by substance-using caregivers have a higher risk of experiencing abuse and neglect (Sagatun-Edwards & Saylor, 2000). In the United States, between 40 and 80% of child maltreatment cases involve parental substance use (Chuang et al., 2012; Lloyd et al., 2017; Testa & Smith, 2009). Such cases may come to the dependency court's attention, and these courts may remove dependents from the home to protect children from harm. Removing children from their parents' guardianship is called out-of-home placement and often takes the form of foster care. More numerous than mental health issues, parental incarceration, and home instability, parental substance use is the most frequent reason for dependency court out-of-home placements (Nicholson, 2006). The number of children in foster care due to parental substance use continues to expand in scale; between 2009 and 2014, there was an 8% increase in foster care placements due to parental substance abuse (Young, 2016). This increase is concerning because these youth experience lower parent-child reunification rates and higher rates of permanent separation from their biological family due to parental rights' termination (He et al., 2014). Further, youth in foster care placement whose parents have substance abuse problems are more likely to become involved in the criminal justice system; this population is known as crossover youth (Herz et al., 2019).

There is some preliminary evidence that growing rates of substance misuse in the United States have a two-fold impact on the child welfare system. Besides the obvious problem of child maltreatment attributable to parent drug and alcohol use, escalating substance use disorder rates in the general population makes recruiting and retaining suitable foster parents even more challenging than it has been previously (Radel et al., 2018). Areas of the U.S. hit particularly hard by substance misuse, particularly opioids, are seeing acute problems in the child welfare system, even when, nationally, the number of children in foster care has declined in some jurisdictions, indicating that parental substance misuse/addiction is driving out-of-home placements (Ghertner et al., 2018; Radel et al., 2018).

Expediting permanency through the Adoption and Safe Families Act (ASFA) of 1997

A permanency plan is developed, and permanent housing placement options pursued (broadly termed "permanency") when parent-child reunification, a type of permanency, fails, and parental rights are terminated. Permanency courses of action include adoption (kinship or nonrelative), long-term foster care, and transfer of legal custody/legal guardianship (Wattenberg et al., 2001). Upwards of 63% of children do not have a permanency plan at the time of parental rights termination. This is not only disruptive to the child; without a permanency plan, children remain in the dependency court workflow, contributing to the dependency court workload (Wattenberg et al., 2001). Dependency court guidelines developed from the Adoption and Safe Families Act (ASFA) of 1997 sought to improve the permanency plan process. Guidelines seek to reduce time in out-of-home placement, expedite permanency outcomes, and ease the court system's burdens. ASFA encouraged timely permanency decisions.

Although the ASFA was initially viewed as a seismic shift to the adoption process nationally, de-emphasizing parent-child reunification and focusing on permanency, there is no substantial evidence that the average speed of adoptions increased since the ASFA's passage (Wulczyn et al.,

2006). To meet these new expediency goals, ASFA promulgated a policy terminating parental rights for children who have been in out-of-home placements for 15 of the most recent 22 months, paving the way for permanent housing placement, expedited case processing, and decreased time to permanency. Under this provision, parents who wish to regain custody of their children have as few as 15-months to demonstrate they are substantially improving the conditions that led to their removal. The policy has led to an increase in the termination of parental rights and out-of-home adoptions. In 1998, the year after ASFA began, the rate of parental rights termination was 10.7%; a decade later, it was 16.2% (U.S. Department of Health and Human Services et al., 2013).

The ASFA policy and its focus on expedited permanency create considerable pressure on parents with substance use disorders, the most common reason for out-of-home placements. It is well documented that achieving sobriety may take multiple attempts, and maintenance can require a continuous approach (Goodson et al., 2020; Manuel et al., 2017). Under the 15-month rule, parents with a drug or alcohol problem have a finite time to achieve sobriety and risk termination of their parental rights if they cannot meet this parent-child reunification requirement. Lercara (2016) suggests that ASFA involves an inappropriate push for adoption; ASFA's 15-month rule may also inhibit parent-child reunification for youth involved with the dependency court because of parental substance use. While ASFA designated this window to reunification with parents, permanency solutions can stretch far longer than this time frame, and children can remain in foster care for a longer period if another permanency solution cannot be realized (Edwards, 2013). Granting courts the authority to terminate parental rights in an accelerated fashion, particularly when substance misuse issues are involved, can have their own negative consequences on children, both in the short-term and as adults, as well as on the parents whose rights are being terminated. This effect can be especially pronounced in underrepresented and underserved communities (Harp & Oser, 2018).

The high stakes of parental sobriety

Before ASFA, parent-child reunification was the permanency goal of dependency courts. Parent-child reunification can only occur if the dependency court determines that court-ordered requirements are met, and parental sobriety is a large component of requirements for cases involving parental substance use. Judges may require parents to receive a level of care assessment, obtain and follow through with all recommendations from a drug and alcohol evaluation, comply with drug and alcohol counseling, and submit to random drug tests. Child welfare caseworkers obtain evaluations and reports from drug and alcohol treatment providers to measure abstinence and treatment adherence. Parent-child reunification typically occurs once dependency courts determine that requirements are met, and it is safe for the child to return home. The pursuit of other permanency outcomes, including parental rights termination, occurs if parent-child reunification is not possible because the parent has not met mandated requirements or home conditions remain unsafe.

Parental substance use is the most common reason for parental rights termination (Wattenberg et al., 2001). Harris-McKoy and colleagues (2014) highlight two important considerations for determining whether it is appropriate to pursue termination of parental rights in cases involving substance abuse: 1) length of time before beginning treatment and 2) progress made in treatment. The 15-month time constraint promulgated by ASFA limits the amount of time in which parents must receive substance abuse treatment and achieve sobriety before a permanency outcome decision is required (Moye & Rinker, 2002). Recovery from addiction is not a straightforward, quick, and easy process, and ASFA's emphasis on expedited permanency may be of significant concern for parents struggling with substance abuse. ASFA's 15-month time limit for permanency outcomes may prove too short for parents to locate and utilize substance abuse services. Several factors, such as insurance approvals, lack of treatment facilities, financial resources, and the wait for an available treatment spot, can affect treatment access (Harris-McKoy et al., 2014). Rockhill et al. (2007) found, on average, that it took almost three months for women to access substance abuse services. Even with an adequate treatment network, it can take longer than 15 months to overcome substance use addictions (Moye & Rinker, 2002). Sobriety can depend on several factors, such as the type of substance used, the severity of use at treatment intake, and treatment modality (Johnson et al., 2020). More time in treatment does lead to fewer relapses though the path to sobriety varies depending on drug choice and length of drug use; simply put, sobriety can take years to achieve and longer to maintain (Sack, 2012). Substance abuse often co-occurs with other problems such as mental health conditions, poor health, poverty, and a general lack of resources and human capital and anxiety over separation from children, further complicating efforts toward parent-child reunification (Priester et al., 2016; Seay et al., 2017). Complex cases where parents have more than one obstacle to reunification to overcome are less likely to result in reunification (Goemans et al., 2016).

There are several factors associated with poorer prospects of reunification once children are placed in out-of-home care. These include being a member of a racial or ethnic minority group (Courtney, 1994, 2000; McDonald et al., 2007), daughters compared to sons (Choi & Ryan, 2007; Landers et al., 2017), younger children (Green et al., 2007; 2008; Sieger, 2020), and length of time spent in out-of-home care (Neil et al., 2020). More than half of children in foster care have siblings and it is important to consider whether there are multiple children from the same parent(s) in out-of-home placement, and the impact this may have on reunification (Guo & Wells, 2003; Shlonsky et al., 2003).

The current study

This study seeks to assess the impact of the ASFA 15-month rule on children's permanency outcomes among children placed in out-of-home care. Our approach is two-pronged. Using logistic regression, we first examine whether there are differences in permanency outcomes across the various circumstances that lead to out-of-home placements. We hypothesize that children in out-of-home placement due to parental substance use or parental substance use plus other types of child abuse/neglect will be less likely to be reunited with their parents than children in out-of-home placement due to non-substance use child abuse/neglect.

Next, we explore whether child characteristics influence parent-child reunification based on the reason for out-of-home placement. Drawing on the literature, we hypothesize that some children have different parent-child reunification prospects based on demographics. We expect Black, Hispanic, female, younger children, and those with siblings in out-of-home placements to be less likely to be reunified with their parents.

A final logistic regression model tests whether the reason for out-of-home placement influences parent-child reunification, controlling for each child's characteristics. We expect children in out-of-home placement due to parental substance use or parental substance use plus other types of child abuse/neglect will be significant predictors of parent-child reunification when child characteristics are added to the model.

Our two-pronged approach's second arm is a set of analyses focusing on the number of days until a permanency decision. Because of the 15-month constraint placed on parent-child reunification by ASFA, we explore which factors contribute to the length of time a child is in out-of-home care. We expect that children in out-of-home placements for a longer period will be less likely to experience reunification with their parents. This analysis is a test of the ASFA goal of any permanency placement compared to parent-child reunification, which was the juvenile dependency courts' original goal before ASFA.

Method

Participants

Data for this study come from the Offices of York County (PA) Children, Youth, and Families and include information on all youth placed in out-of-home care through the York County dependency court between January 1, 2015, and February 28, 2017 ($N = 558$). The Offices of York (PA) County Children, Youth, and Families work in tandem with the county's dependency court to support child welfare and track out-of-home placements and permanency outcomes. We followed all cases until December 31, 2018, allowing at least 22 months of follow-up after child placement in out-of-home care. ASFA requires states to pursue parental rights termination for children who have been in out-of-home care for 15 of the past 22 months.

The administrative data were deidentified before it was received. This research was reviewed and approved by the Pennsylvania State University's Institutional Review Board and waiver to the consent process was granted.

Dependent variables

Parent-child reunification

The study's focus is on permanency outcomes for the child. There are four possible permanency outcomes for children who experience an out-of-home placement through the dependency court: (1) parent-child reunification; (2) adoption; (3) transfer of legal custody/legal guardianship; and (4) living with other relatives. For this study, parent-child reunification is the main dependent variable; it is coded as 1 = *parent-child reunification* and 0 = *other permanency outcome.*

Time to permanency outcome

A continuous variable denotes the number of days in out-of-home care counted from the first day of out-of-home placement to either parent-child reunification, other permanency outcomes, or the end-of-study period. We calculate the time to permanency variable as the day the child began their out-of-home placement until they received a permanency outcome. Youth who had not yet achieved a permanency outcome before the end of the data collection period, December 31, 2018, were right-censored ($n = 21$).

Independent variable

Reason leading to out-of-home-placement

The main predictor variable of interest is parental substance use as the circumstance leading to out-of-home placement. Other possible circumstances included physical abuse, sexual abuse, neglect, abandonment, and child's behavior. A nominal variable was created to capture three reasons leading to out-of-home placement: 1) parental substance use only; 2) parental substance use plus other types of child abuse/neglect (e.g., physical abuse, sexual abuse, neglect, and parental incarceration); and 3) child abuse/neglect reasons other than substance use.

Control variables

For some analyses, we include controls that may influence permanency outcomes. We include dummy variables for child's race (*white*, *Black*, *Other*) and ethnicity (1 = *Hispanic* or 0 = *non-Hispanic*), a dichotomous measure of sex (1 = *male*, 0 = *female*), and a continuous measure of the child's age at the time of out-of-home placement plus a categorical grouping of age (0-4, 5-7, 8-11, 12-15, and 16-19). We also created a dummy variable to identify whether a child was a member of a sibling group where multiple children were placed in out-of-home care through the juvenile dependency court, where 1 = *multiple children were removed from the home* and 0 = *only one child was removed from the home.*

Analytical plan

We employ multiple statistical techniques using STATA 16 to test study hypotheses. Descriptive statistics were generated for all variables. Logistic regression for binary outcome variables is used for models when parent-child reunification is the dependent variable. Using a Cox proportional hazard model (Cox, 1972) and Kaplan-Meier survival analysis, we then examine whether the time to permanency outcome is longer for youth in the dependency court due to parental substance use. A Cox proportional hazard model assesses the time to permanency outcome, a continuous variable. A Cox proportional hazard model is a type of semi-parametric hazard model used when the hazard ratio for two subgroups is constant over a period of time. This model will determine time to an event (permanency outcome) while controlling for variables that may influence that event's timing. Kaplan-Meier survival analysis (Kaplan & Meier, 1958) is used to visually compare two survival curves depicting time to event (in this study, parent-child reunification), and a log-rank test quantifies any difference in time. Only two variables, race and ethnicity, had missing data. The percentage of missing data was low (< 5%), and therefore stepwise deletion was employed.

Results

Descriptive statistics

Table 1 displays the sample's descriptive statistics, which was processed by the York County juvenile dependency court between January 1, 2015, and February 28, 2017. Most children processed through the York County juvenile dependency court during this period were reunited with their parents (*N*=334, 59.86%). In contrast to the literature on factors impacting out-of-home placements, most children who came to this court's attention were placed in out-of-home care due to abuse/neglect reasons that did not include substance use (*N*=360, 64.52%). Children in the juvenile dependency court with out-of-home placements due to parental substance use comprised 17.03% of the sample, and children with out-of-home placements due to parental substance use plus other child abuse/neglect types made up 18.46%.

Table 1. Descriptive statistics for youth in out-of-home placements in the York county dependency court, January 1, 2015 – February 28, 2017.

Variable	Coding	N	%
Dependent Variable			
Permanency outcome	Parent-child reunification = 1	334	59.86
	Other permanency outcome = 0	203	36.38
	Case right censored	21	3.76
Independent Variable			
Reason for out-of-home placement	Parental substance use only	95	17.03
	Parental substance use plus other types of child abuse/neglect	103	18.46
	Other types of child abuse/neglect	360	64.52
Youth Characteristics			
Race	White	378	68.11
	Black	132	23.78
	Other	45	8.11
Ethnicity	Hispanic = 1	80	14.57
	Non-Hispanic = 0	469	85.43
Gender	Male = 1	286	51.25
	Female = 0	272	48.76
Multiple children removed from home	Yes = 1	310	55.56
	No = 0	248	44.44
Age group at placement	0-4	102	18.28
	5-7	76	13.62
	8-11	63	11.29
	12-15	84	15.05
	16-19	233	41.76
		M	**SD**
Age	Continuous variable (0-19)	6.43	5.58
Length of care (days)	Continuous variable (1-1,337)	203.16	238.28

Most children were white ($N = 378$, 68.11%) and non-Hispanic ($N = 469$, 85.43%) which is representative of the county's demographic characteristics. Boys comprised just more than half of the children ($N = 286$; 51.25%), and 55.56% ($N = 310$) of children had siblings also in out-of-home placement. The average age of children in the juvenile dependency court at the time of their placement in out-of-home care during the study period was 6.43 years, with participants ranging from less than one-year-old to 19 years old. The average length of time a child was in out-of-home placement was for less than one year ($M = 203.16$ days, SD = 238.28).

Multinomial logistic regression

A series of multivariate logistic regression models examine predictors of parent-child reunification (Table 2). The first model shows that out-of-home placement due to substance use plus other types of child neglect/abuse is significantly associated with a reduced likelihood of parent-child reunification ($\beta = -.87$, $p = .000$) compared to children in out-of-home placements due to other types of child abuse/neglect. The second model shows that Black children are more likely than whites to be reunited with their parents ($\beta = .47$, $p = .041$). Parent-child reunification is also more likely among older children ($\beta = .06$, $p = .001$). Children with siblings who are also in out-of-home placement are less likely to be reunited with their parents ($\beta = -.46$, $p = .018$).

In the full regression model (Table 2, Model 3), the most notable finding is that out-of-home placement for parental substance abuse only, which approached significance at the 95% level of confidence in Model 1 is not significant. In Model 1, children with out-of-home placements due to substance use plus other types of child abuse/neglect were significantly less likely to be reunited with their parents, and this relationship remains

Table 2. Predictors of parent-child reunification.

	Model 1		Model 2		Model 3	
	β (SE)	*p*-value	β (SE)	*p*-value	β (SE)	*p*-value
Out-of-home placement due to parental substance use only	−.43 (.24)	0.072			-.07 (.26)	0.780
Out-of-home placement due to substance use plus other types of child abuse/neglect	−.87 (.23)	0.000			-.63 (.24)	0.010
Black			.47 (.23)	0.041	.39 (.24)	0.103
Other race			.41 (.35)	0.236	.39 (.35)	0.264
Hispanic origin			.17 (.27)	0.541	.12 (.28)	0.675
Male			.04 (.18)	0.820	.08 (.19)	0.674
Age at out-of-home placement			.06 (.02)	0.001	.05 (.02)	0.004
Multiple children removed from home			-.46 (.19)	0.018	-.42 (.19)	0.030

Note: The referent categories are out-of-home placement due to other types of child abuse/neglect and white.

Table 3. Hazard ratio and 95% confidence intervals (CI) of time to parent-child reunification permanency outcome by risk factor, among youth placed in out-of-home care through the York county dependency court between January 1, 2015 and February 28, 2017 (N = 558).

	Hazard ratio (95% confidence interval)	*p*-value
Out-of-home placement due to parental substance use only	0.94 (0.68, 1.29)	0.705
Out-of-home placement due to substance use plus other types of child neglect/abuse	0.65 (0.47, 0.89)	0.009
Black	1.26 (0.97, 1.65)	0.085
Other race	1.21 (0.82, 1.81)	0.337
Hispanic origin	0.97 (0.71, 1.31)	0.830
Male	0.99 (0.71, 1.31)	0.931
Age at out-of-home placement	1.03 (1.01, 1.05)	0.006
Multiple children removed from home	0.75 (0.59, 0.94)	0.013

significant in Model 3, which controls for child demographics. Age at time of out-of-home placement remains a significant predictor of parent-child reunification (β = .05, p = .004), meaning older children are more likely to be reunited with parents, and having siblings in out-of-home placement decreases a child's chance of returning home (β = –.42, p = .030).

Cox proportional hazard model

In the Cox proportional hazard model (Table 3), the outcome of interest is time until a parent-child permanency outcome. Hazard ratios depict the probability that an individual at time t realizes a given event (parent-child reunification) by the end of the study period and the rate at which the event of interest occurred. Hazard ratios can be interpreted as odds ratios in logistic regression. A hazard ratio of 1 is interpreted as no difference, a hazard ratio greater than 1 means there is increased risk between groups, and a hazard below 1 indicates decreased risk. An increased risk means children were in out-of-home placement longer, while a decreased risk indicates a permanency decision was reached sooner. For continuous variables, the percent change is calculated as $100[\exp(\beta)-1]$, or more simply, 100*(HR-1), where HR = hazard ratio.

The parent-child reunification rate of children placed in out-of-home care due to parental substance use plus other types of child abuse/neglect drops by 35% compared to children in out-of-home placement for reasons that do not include substance use. Parent-child reunification rates among children with siblings in out-of-home placement are three-quarters those of children without siblings in out-of-home care. The odds of parent-child reunification are 3% higher with each increase in age category.

Kaplan-Meier survival analysis

Figure 1 portrays survival curves of time until permanency placement outcome. Using a log-rank test (χ^2 = 122.02, p = .000), we see a

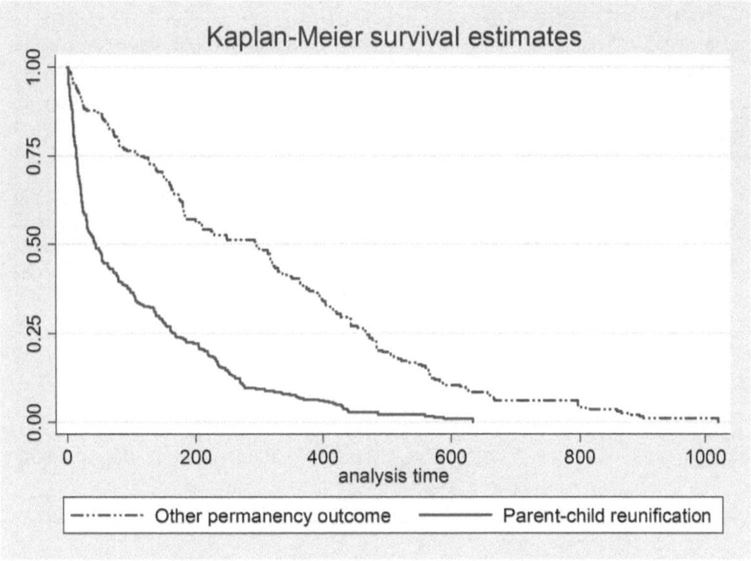

Figure 1. Kaplan-Meier survival, time to permanency outcome among youth placed in out-of-home care through the York county dependency court between January 1, 2015 and February 28, 2017 ($N=558$).

statistically significant difference in time to permanency placement for parent-child reunification compared to other permanency outcomes.

Time to permanency outcome for the three significant predictors identified in the proportional hazard model is also tested. Log-rank tests stratified by out-of-home placement due to parental substance use plus other types of child abuse/neglect (χ^2 = 11.71, p = .0006; Figure 2), age group at placement (χ^2 = 5.43, p = .143; survival curve not shown), and having siblings also in out-of-home placement (χ^2 = 15.76, p = .0001; Figure 3) visually demonstrate how these two predictor variables influence time to permanency outcomes.

Discussion

The Adoption and Safe Families Act (ASFA) encourages decisions on permanency within an expedited timeframe by stressing the health and safety of the child as a paramount concern, and to this end provides both mandatory and optional directives to the states for expedited termination of parental rights (Hort, 2000). ASFA obligates states to begin termination of parental rights proceedings when a child has been in out-of-home care for 15 of the last 22 months. ASFA allows concurrent planning in which efforts at parent-child reunification proceed simultaneously with attempts to achieve alternative permanency such as legal guardianship or adoption. Lercara (2016) proposes that ASFA be amended to put more of an emphasis

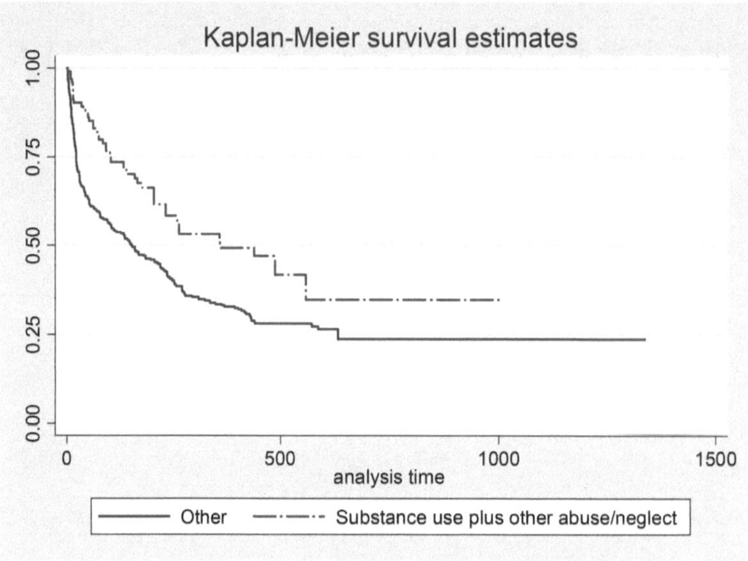

Figure 2. Kaplan-Meier survival, time to permanency outcome among youth placed in out-of-home care due to parental substance use plus other abuse/neglect.

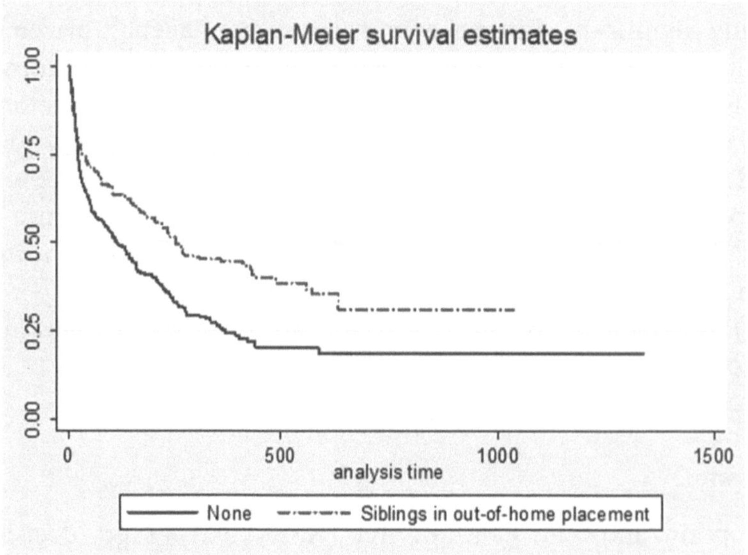

Figure 3. Kaplan-Meier survival, time to permanency outcome stratified by siblings in out-of-home placement.

on reuniting children back with his/her natural parents. This study identifies key factors associated with successful parent-child reunification in a timely manner. In the study setting, it appears a more enlightened approach is taken toward parents whose maltreatment of their children stems solely from substance misuse issues. The analyses indicate parental substance misuse, by itself, is not typically grounds for terminating parental rights, and that reunification for such households is a primary focus with the 22-month window outlined by ASFA.

The results also demonstrate potential areas of concern for reunification. When younger children are removed from the home, the data indicate that parental rights termination is more likely than when a child is removed from the home at an older age. It may be that agencies are less concerned with parental reunification of younger children because of the higher likelihood of another desirable permanency outcome such as adoption. Similarly, termination of parental rights for older children may be slower if a permanency solution is unlikely to occur, subjecting the child to more time in temporary placement in the foster care system. Also, children with siblings in out-of-home placement are significantly less likely to be reunified, which is a troubling finding if the study jurisdiction is representative of other jurisdictions. Most children in the sample (55.6%) had siblings removed from parental custody. A different permanency outcome may be preferable in such situations due to the alterations parents must make to ensure their home is suitable for reunification with multiple children.

Further, such families may have younger children whose permanency scenarios may look very different from their older siblings. Future research must look into the intricacies of permanency outcomes for parents with substance use disorders who have multiple children in the dependency court system, so it can be determined which factors play the greatest role in reunification or another permanency outcome for each child in the family. Scholars should also examine the parent-child reunification process for families with multiple children in different foster care situations (e.g., sibling groups placed together in foster homes compared to siblings living in multiple foster homes). This study was unable to address this important aspect of reunification because data on foster care placements for sibling groups were not available for analysis.

ASFA provides financial inducements to states that accomplish a successful foster care adoption. All states are granted a base number for the estimated amount of foster care adoptions they should have within the fiscal year. A state is awarded $4,000 for each additional foster child adopted and receives an additional incentive for placing a foster care child up for adoption. For a state to receive the incentives, ASFA requires the state to file a petition to terminate the natural parents' rights if reunification has not been successful within 15 months. With these financial incentives in play, Lercara (2016) points out that it may often be easier to find state agencies putting their own best interests before the best interest of a child. Although the present research findings are preliminary, it does not appear that agencies in the study jurisdiction have used the provisions specified in ASFA to benefit financially or in any other way. The data indicate that children in the study jurisdiction are reunified with parents as often as is feasible, with only the most problematic cases resulting in another permanent or temporary placement option. However, the ASFA 15-month ruling may unintentionally disrupt the adoption process. Coakley and Berrick (2008, p. 110) aptly state that "It is unrealistic to expect that any policy or practice could eliminate the chance of adoption disruption." Additional work is needed to understand if the parental sobriety requirement under ASFA places undue pressure on the reunification process and contributes failed adoptions.

County social services agencies must provide 'reasonable efforts' at reunification and include counseling, substance abuse treatment, parenting assessment, home-based services, domestic violence treatment, and transportation. The subjective nature of the reasonable efforts coupled with the financial incentives provided to states placing children into adoptive homes, can effectively undermine the goal of reunification (Lercara, 2016). This is often a result of aggravating circumstances that allow states not to make reasonable efforts to reunify the child with his/her natural parents. Lercara proposes that ASFA be amended to replace the term 'reasonable efforts' with the term 'best efforts.' Having a best-efforts standard would increase the child welfare agency's obligation to work toward the permanency goal of reunifying the family, even if that prolongs time in the juvenile dependency court. While it is certain that a number, likely a majority, of child welfare agencies in the U.S. (including the study locale) adhere to a de facto 'best efforts' standard toward the goal of restoring parental custody of children in the system, there may be jurisdictions that see parental reunification as unlikely or even detrimental to the well-being of the child or children involved. Thus, the financial and time incentive of ASFA may actually end up working counter to family reunification as a permanency solution.

Limitations

This study is not without limitations. The generalizability of these results is subject to certain constraints. For instance, the study area is limited to one large county in a northeastern state. While the study location does encompass rural, suburban, and urban areas, it is limited in its racial and ethnic diversity. According to the 2010 Census, the population was 88.7% white, 7.1% Black, and 8.1% Hispanic (U.S. Census, 2021). Notwithstanding these limitations, the study adds to our understanding of the child permanency process under ASFA. While the study did not evaluate what types of child abuse/neglect beyond substance use (e.g., physical abuse, sexual abuse, parental incarceration) may have contributed to permanency outcomes because of small sample sizes of these different case circumstances, its findings highlight their amplified effect on parent-child reunification. Future research should aim greater focus on the effect of parental substance use plus other child abuse/neglect on parent-child reunification. Such work could produce interesting findings that account for more nuanced implications of ASFA on time to permanency among parents whose juvenile dependency court cases present with multiple child maltreatment concerns. Research into this area is an essential next step in confirming the present study's findings and addressing its limitations.

Practical implications

Permanency for young children removed due to parental drug use often occurs at two levels. The first level suggests that younger children are more likely to be adopted than older children leading to dependency courts having a higher sense of comfort in terminating parental rights given that permanency is the goal under ASFA (Akin, 2011; Connell et al., 2006). The second level suggests that parents who have had multiple children removed from their care are perhaps seen as less likely to successfully address both substance misuse and other factors which led to separation from their children, therefore other permanency solutions apart from reunification were pursued by agencies within the timeframe established by ASFA. This study was unable to address sibling group placement and whether siblings were placed together or reunified at the same time. Future research in multiple settings should examine whether these factors impact permanency decisions in any appreciable manner. For example, is parental reunification more likely if children from the same family are in separate placements? Similarly, will other, more expedient, permanency outcomes be pursued when siblings are placed together, and that setting is an option for permanent placement?

Quick and easy access into treatment programs and successful completion of at least one program can increase the likelihood of reunification. In return, the amount of time a child spends in out-of-home placements decreases (He et al., 2014), a desirable outcome for the family and the various social agencies involved. Choi (2019) encourages more timely treatment access while also highlighting the need for recovery coaches to supplement treatment efforts. Targeting parents with younger children removed from the home, multiple children in the system, and co-occurring child endangerment issues and substance abuse will likely help limited agency resources have a greater impact than treating all substance misusing parents in the same manner. Barriers to treatment, substance misuse, and otherwise, remain a persistent issue in underserved communities (Mennis et al., 2012; Pullen & Oser, 2014). The study setting fits this description, both socio-economically and geographically. In 2017, Pennsylvania's death rate by illicit narcotics (44.3 per 100,000) was the third worst in the nation (Kawasaki et al., 2019). Compounding the issue, in mid-year 2018, there were 24 providers of buprenorphine treatment within a 25-mile radius of the city of Harrisburg, which was the same ($n = 24$) number of those within a 50-mile radius of Harrisburg (Kawasaki et al., 2019). York is 26.3 miles from Harrisburg, indicating that services outside the state capital in less populated areas of the state are scarce, even with documented growth in substance misuse in the overall population. In the end, parents in York County who desire to address their substance misuse issues and work toward reunification with their children must do so with limited access to resources that could assist them to those ends.

Acknowledgments

We are grateful to the Offices of York County (PA) Children, Youth, and Families for providing access to the dataset used in this study.

Disclosure statement

Mitra Honardoost is employed by the Offices of York County (PA) Children, Youth, and Families. Eileen M. Ahlin and Don Hummer declare that they have no conflicts to report.

Ethical standards and informed consent

All procedures followed were in accordance with the ethical standards of the responsible committee on human experimentation at the Pennsylvania State University and with the Helsinki Declaration of 1975, as revised in 2000. Informed consent was waived; the secondary dataset did not contain identifying information.

ORCID

Eileen M. Ahlin http://orcid.org/0000-0002-1604-2657

References

Akin, B. A. (2011). Predictors of foster care exits to permanency: A competing risks analysis of reunification, guardianship, and adoption. *Children and Youth Services Review*, *33*(6), 999–1011. https://doi.org/10.1016/j.childyouth.2011.01.008

Choi, S., & Ryan, J. P. (2007). Co-occurring problems for substance abusing mothers in child welfare: Matching services to improve family reunification. *Children and Youth Services Review*, *29*(11), 1395–1410. https://doi.org/10.1016/j.childyouth.2007.05.013

Choi, S., (2019). Improving children-parents visitation for families with substance abuse problems in child welfare. *Journal of Social Science for Policy Implications*, *7*(1), 1–6.

Chuang, E., Moore, K., Barrett, B., & Young, M. S. (2012). Effect of an integrated family dependency treatment court on child welfare reunification, time to permanency and re-entry rates. *Children and Youth Services Review*, *34*(9), 1896–1902. https://doi.org/10.1016/j.childyouth.2012.06.001

Coakley, J. F., & Berrick, J. D. (2008). Research review: In a rush to permanency: Preventing adoption disruption. *Child and Family Social Work*, *13*(1), 101–112.

Connell, C. M., Katz, K. H., Saunders, L., & Tebes, J. K. (2006). Leaving foster care—The influence of child and case characteristics on foster care exit rates. *Children and Youth Services Review*, *28*(7), 780–798. https://doi.org/10.1016/j.childyouth.2005.08.007

Courtney, M. E. (1994). Factors associated with the reunification of foster children with their families. *Social Service Review*, *68*(1), 81–108. https://doi.org/10.1086/604034

Courtney, M. E. (2000). Research needed to improve the prospects for children in out-of-home placement. *Children and Youth Services Review*, *22*(9-10), 743–761. https://doi.org/10.1016/S0190-7409(00)00115-8

Cox, D. R. (1972). Regression models and life-tables (with discussion). *Journal of the Royal Statistical Society*, *34*(2), 187–220.

Edwards, H. R. (2013). A profile of post-ASFA hearings in the U.S. Congress. *Child Welfare*, *92*(1), 65–88.

Ghertner, R., Waters, A., Radel, L., & Crouse, G. (2018). The role of substance use in child welfare caseloads. *Children and Youth Services Review*, *90*, 83–93. https://doi.org/10.1016/j.childyouth.2018.05.015

Goemans, A., Vanderfaeillie, J., Damen, H., Pijnenburg, H., & Van Holen, F. (2016). Reunification of foster children: Factors associated with reunification outcomes in Flanders and the Netherlands. *Children and Youth Services Review*, *70*, 284–292. https://doi.org/10.1016/j.childyouth.2016.09.023

Goodson, M. V., Morash, M., & Kashy, D. A. (2020). The moderating effect of substance abuse treatment engagement on the connection between support from program participants and substance-related recidivism for justice-involved women. *International Journal of Offender Therapy and Comparative Criminology*, *64*(12), 1217–1235. https://doi.org/10.1177/0306624X19863218

Green, B. L., Rockhill, A., & Burrus, S. (2008). The role of interagency collaboration for substance-abusing families involved with child welfare. *Child Welfare*, *87*(1), 29–61.

Green, B. L., Rockhill, A., & Furrer, C. (2007). Does substance abuse treatment make a difference for child welfare case outcomes? A statewide longitudinal analysis. *Children and Youth Services Review*, *29*(4), 460–473. https://doi.org/10.1016/j.childyouth.2006.08.006

Guo, S., & Wells, K. (2003). Research on timing of foster care outcomes: Methodological problems and approaches. *Social Service Review*, *77*(1), 1–24. https://doi.org/10.1086/345702

Harp, K. L. H., & Oser, C. B. (2018). A longitudinal analysis of the impact of child custody loss on drug use and crime among a sample of African American mothers. *Child Abuse & Neglect*, *77*, 1–12. https://doi.org/10.1016/j.chiabu.2017.12.017

Harris-McKoy, D., Meyer, A. S., McWey, L. M., & Henderson, T. L. (2014). Substance use, policy, and foster care. *Journal of Family Issues*, *35*(10), 1298–1321. https://doi.org/10.1177/0192513X13481439

He, A. S., Traube, D. E., & Young, N. K. (2014). Perceptions of parental substance use disorders in cross-system collaboration among child welfare, alcohol and other drugs, and dependency court organizations. *Child Abuse & Neglect*, *38*(5), 939–951. https://doi.org/10.1016/j.chiabu.2013.10.020

Herz, D. C., Dierkhising, C. B., Raithel, J., Schretzman, M., Guiltinan, S., Goerge, R. M., Cho, Y., Coulton, C., & Abbott, S. (2019). Dual system youth and their pathways: A comparison of incidence, characteristics and system experiences using linked administrative data. *Journal of Youth and Adolescence*, *48*(12), 2432–2450. https://doi.org/10.1007/s10964-019-01090-3

Hort, K. A. (2000). Is twenty-two months beyond the best interest of the child? ASFA's guidelines for the termination of parental rights. *Fordham Urban Law Journal*, *28*, 1879–1922.

Johnson, K., Rigg, K. K., & Eyles, C. H. (2020). Receiving addiction treatment in the US: Do patient demographics, drug of choice, or substance use disorder severity matter?*International Journal of Drug Policy*, *75*. https://doi.org/10.1016/j.drugpo.2019.10.009

Kaplan, E. L., & Meier, P. (1958). Nonparametric estimation from incomplete observations. *Journal of the American Statistical Association*, *53*(282), 457–481. https://doi.org/10.1080/01621459.1958.10501452

Kawasaki, S., Francis, E., Mills, S., Buchberger, G., Hogentogler, R., & Kraschnewski, J. (2019). Multi-model implementation of evidence-based care in the treatment of opioid use disorder in Pennsylvania. *Journal of Substance Abuse Treatment*, *106*, 58–64. https://doi.org/10.1016/j.jsat.2019.08.016

Landers, A. L., Danes, S. M., Harstad, J., & Hawk, S. W. (2017). Finding their way home: Factors associated with reunification for American Indian and White adults. *Children and Youth Services Review*, *82*, 359–364. https://doi.org/10.1016/j.childyouth.2017.09.002

Lercara, B. (2016). The adoption and safe families act: Proposing a "best efforts" standard to eliminate the ultimate obstacle for parent-child reunification. *Family Court Review*, *54*(4), 657–670. https://doi.org/10.1111/fcre.12250

Lloyd, M. H., Akin, B. A., & Brook, J. (2017). Parental drug use and permanency for young children in foster care: A competing risks analysis of reunification, guardianship, and adoption. *Children and Youth Services Review*, *77*(C), 177–187. https://doi.org/10.1016/j.childyouth.2017.04.016

Manuel, J. I., Yuan, Y., Herman, D. B., Svikis, D. S., Nichols, O., Palmer, E., & Deren, S. (2017). Barriers and facilitators to successful transition from long-term residential substance abuse treatment. *Journal of Substance Abuse Treatment*, *74*, 16–22. https://doi.org/10.1016/j.jsat.2016.12.001

McDonald, T. P., Poertner, J., & Jennings, M. A. (2007). Permanency for children in foster care: A competing risks analysis. *Journal of Social Service Research*, *33*(4), 45–56. https://doi.org/10.1300/J079v33n04_04

Mennis, J., Stahler, G. J., & Baron, D. A. (2012). Geographic barriers to community-based psychiatric treatment for drug-dependent patients. *Annals of the Association of American Geographers*, *102*(5), 1093–1103. https://doi.org/10.1080/00045608.2012.657142

Moye, J., & Rinker, R. (2002). It's a hard knock life: Does the Adoption and Safe Families Act of 1997 adequately address problems in the child welfare system?*Harvard Journal on Legislation*, *39*, 375–394.

Neil, E., Gitsels, L., & Thoburn, J. (2020). Returning children home from care: What can be learned from local authority data?*Child & Family Social Work*, *25*(3), 548–556. https://doi.org/10.1111/cfs.12724

Nicholson, E. K. (2006). Racing against the ASFA clock: How incarcerated parents lose more than freedom. *Duquesne Law Review*, *45*(1), 83–95.

Priester, M. A., Browne, T., Iachini, A., Clone, S., DeHart, D., & Seay, K. D. (2016). Treatment access barriers and disparities among individuals with co-occurring mental health and substance use disorders: An integrative literature review. *Journal of Substance Abuse Treatment*, *61*, 47–59. https://doi.org/10.1016/j.jsat.2015.09.006

Pullen, E., & Oser, C. (2014). Barriers to Substance abuse treatment in rural and urban communities: Counselor perspectives. *Substance Use & Misuse*, *49*(7), 891–901. https://doi.org/10.3109/10826084.2014.891615

Radel, L., Baldwin, M., Crouse, G., Ghertner, R., Waters, A. (2018). *Substance use, the opioid epidemic, and the child welfare system: Key findings from a mixed methods study.* ASPE Research Brief, U.S. Department of Health & Human Services, Office of the Assistant Secretary for Planning and Evaluation. Retrieved from: https://aspe.hhs.gov/system/files/pdf/258836/SubstanceUseChildWelfareOverview.pdf

Rockhill, A., Green, B. L., & Furrer, C. (2007). Is the adoption and safe families act influencing child welfare outcomes for families with substance abuse issues?*Child Maltreatment*, *12*(1), 7–19. https://doi.org/10.1177/1077559506296139

Sack, D. (2012). How long does addiction recovery take?*Psych Central*. https://psychcentral.com/blog/addiction-recovery/2012/01/how-long-addiction-recovery#1

Sagatun-Edwards, I., & Saylor, C. (2000). A coordinated approach to improving outcomes for substance-abusing families in juvenile dependency court. *Juvenile and Family Court Journal*, *51*(4), 1–16. https://doi.org/10.1111/j.1755-6988.2000.tb00028.x

Seay, K. D., Iachini, A. L., DeHart, D. D., Browne, T., & Clone, S. (2017). Substance abuse treatment engagement among mothers: Perceptions of the parenting role and agency-related motivators and inhibitors. *Journal of Family Social Work*, *20*(3), 196–212. https://doi.org/10.1080/10522158.2017.1300113

Shlonsky, A., Webster, D., & Needell, B. (2003). The ties that bind: A cross-sectional analysis of siblings in foster care. *Journal of Social Service Research*, *29*(3), 27–52. https://doi.org/10.1300/J079v29n03_02

Sieger, M. H. L. (2020). Reunification for young children of color with substance removals: An intersectional analysis of longitudinal national data. *Child Abuse & Neglect*, *108*. https://doi.org/10.1016/j.chiabu.2020.104664

Testa, M. F., & Smith, B. (2009). Prevention and drug treatment. *The Future of Children*, *19*(2), 147–168.

U.S. Census. (2021). *Quick facts, York County, Pennsylvania*. https://www.census.gov/quickfacts/yorkcountypennsylvania

U.S. Department of Health and Human Services, Administration for Children and Families, & Children's Bureau. (2013). *Child welfare outcomes 2008–2011: Report to congress*. Retrieved from: https://www.acf.hhs.gov/sites/default/files/cb/cwo0811.pdf#page=7

Wattenberg, E., Kelley, M., & Kim, H. (2001). When the rehabilitation ideal fails: A study of parental rights termination. *Child Welfare*, *80*(4), 405–431.

Wulczyn, F. H., Chen, L., & Hislop, K. B. (2006). Adoption dynamics and the Adoption and Safe Families Act. *Social Service Review*, *80*(4), 584–608. https://doi.org/10.1086/508558

Young, N. K. (2016). *Examining the impact of the opioid epidemic. Written testimony*, U.S. Senate Committee on Homeland Security and Governmental Affairs. Retrieved from http://www.cffutures.org/files/Young_Homeland%20Security%20and%20Governmental%20Affairs%20Final.pdf

Reunification, alienation, or re-traumatization? Let's start listening to the child

Suzanne Chester

ABSTRACT
"Reunification therapy" is regularly ordered in family court for children who resist contact with a parent they claim is abusive. Based on my client's experience of court-ordered reunification with her father who had sexually abused her, this case study demonstrates the harmful effect of forced contact between a child and an abusive parent. My client's involvement in this reunification process further illustrates how implicit bias can cause family court professionals to mistakenly attribute a child's legitimate estrangement from a parent to "parental alienation". To prevent further harm to the child, and to ensure that courts receive reliable evidence of the child's experience, this case study highlights the need for the appointment of a trauma-informed attorney to advocate for the child's expressed interests.

In family courts across the United States, children who reject contact with a parent they report is abusive often find themselves in one of three situations: (1) they are ordered to attend unregulated reunification programs with that parent; (2) their custody is abruptly switched to the custody of the parent they reject; or (3) they are ordered to participate in weekly sessions of "reunification therapy." In recent years, researchers have warned of the potentially harmful effects of forcing a child to attend unregulated "reunification camps" where the child is held against their will and pressured to reject the influence of the parent with whom they are most bonded (Dallam & Silberg, 2016; Mercer, 2019). Other writers have cautioned that custody reversals are counterproductive and more likely to reinforce the child's disaffection for the rejected parent (Kelly & Johnston, 2001). Through a series of case studies, Silberg and Dallam (2019) have documented the harm to children when the court did not credit the abuse and placed children in the custody of the abusive parent. Decisions in these cases were later reversed when evidence of abuse was finally credited.

This case study will focus on my client's experience of reunification therapy, arguably the least radical intervention of the three commonly ordered in family courts. I represented twelve-year old Jane (pseudonym to protect child's identity) in a contentious custody case between her parents in which my client had been forced to undergo reunification therapy and supervised visits for eighteen months with her father. Two years after the attempted reunification was terminated, Jane's father filed a motion to resume the process again. At her mother's request, the court appointed The Child's Advocate of Legal Aid of North Carolina to represent Jane, and it was in this capacity that I came to be the child's attorney. Written with the permission of Jane and her mother, this retrospective case study has three objectives: first, to explore the detrimental effects of forced contact between Jane and her father; second, to demonstrate how implicit bias caused family court professionals to mistakenly attribute Jane's legitimate estrangement to "parental alienation." And third, this article argues that children in custody cases involving allegations or evidence of abuse must be appointed a trauma-informed attorney to advocate for their expressed interests. In this way, courts can receive evidence of the child's experience, and minimize the risk of children being harmed by inappropriate reunification efforts.

Many professionals have written about reunification therapy and other interventions for children who resist contact with a parent. (see Fidler et al., 2012 for a review of this literature). More recently, Kleinman (2017) has challenged the ethics and efficacy of reunification therapy. There is a dearth of empirical research published about either the benefits or the potential harms of this intervention. Researchers have underscored the need for establishing independent systems for detecting potentially harmful effects of psychotherapy, noting that case studies that bring to light possible harms are particularly useful for highlighting the need for future research (Dimidjian & Hollon,2010). Mercer (2019) has emphasized the need to pay greater attention to anecdotal accounts of the detrimental effects of a particular mental health intervention, especially when such treatments are court ordered for children who are powerless to refuse them.

Litigation concerning Jane

When I met Jane, she was twelve years old, and her parents had been litigating custody, visitation, abuse, and neglect issues from the time she was born. The litigation took place in the courts of three different states and Child Protective Services ("CPS") agencies in multiple jurisdictions. One of the first legal motions in the case was Jane's mother's request for an emergency order to enable her to breastfeed Jane during her father's visitation—an arrangement agreed to in their separation agreement but later reneged upon by her father. In 2009, when Jane was almost three years old, a report was made to CPS. After an investigation, CPS substantiated that her father had sexually abused her. The father appealed and the decision was reversed by an administrative court on the grounds that CPS had not excluded other potential perpetrators of Jane's abuse. As a toddler, Jane had to be treated for severe allergies to cats and dogs, allergies repeatedly exacerbated by exposure to pets at her father's home. When Jane was four, the court prohibited him from bringing Jane to his home unless he permanently removed all animals from his residence. After moving to North Carolina with her mother, the four-year old child had visitation once a month with her father and his wife in a hotel. After the fourth visit, Jane disclosed to her grandmother that her father had sexually abused her. A report was made to CPS and Jane's mother had to sign a safety plan prohibiting any contact between the child and her father while CPS investigated. The court granted the mother emergency custody of Jane.

The court finds that the four-year old had been sexually abused

Some months later, the court conducted a review of its emergency order. After hearing testimony from the CPS investigator and Jane's individual therapist, the court accepted their conclusion that Jane had been sexually abused by her father, finding that

> the child's reporting of the abuse by the father was spontaneous and consistent yet varied enough so as not to seem coached or robotic, and then when taken together with the minor child's sexual acting out and other behaviors, each professional independently came to the conclusion the child had been sexually abused.

In the same order, referencing the earlier substantiation of sexual abuse in 2009, the court observed that despite the reversal on appeal, the CPS case workers still believed that Jane had been sexually abused. After the hearing, the court noted there was "no credible evidence to support the possibility of a different perpetrator." The court found that Jane's father "refused to accept any responsibility for the current situation and blamed Jane's mother and her family for coaching Jane to report the abuse." The court noted the father had done little to improve his relationship with Jane since the entry of the 2011 emergency order—having failed to obtain the psychological evaluation ordered by the court and having rejected invitations to engage in reunification treatment with the child.

By contrast, the court found that Jane's mother had ensured the minor child was receiving therapy with a therapist she trusted, had obtained her own psychological evaluation, and as recommended by CPS, was receiving her own group and individual therapy for non-offending parents. The court ordered Jane's father not to return to court to request visitation until he had engaged in reunification therapy with his daughter, and Jane's therapist believed it was appropriate for him to have visitation with the child. Two years later, the parents filed motions making starkly divergent claims. Jane's mother stated that Jane's therapist had released the child from treatment because she was asymptomatic and would continue to be on condition that she had no interaction with her father. By contrast, the father alleged that Jane's mother was alienating him from Jane and had frustrated his efforts to start reunification therapy by changing Jane's therapist. He asked the court to hold her in contempt.

The court responds to the father's claims of "parental alienation"

At the next hearing, the same judge found that Jane had been diagnosed with PTSD and had been re-traumatized by attending a child sexual abuse prevention program at her school. Jane's mother brought her to a "trauma specialist" to whom Jane divulged additional details of sexual abuse by her father. Although the father had not had any contact with Jane for more than two years, the trauma specialist made a report to CPS, who, in turn, ordered a comprehensive forensic examination ("CFE") for Jane. The CFE was not a part of the court file, the court made no reference to its findings, and this writer did not have access to it. It was, however, ordered to be provided to the professionals involved in the reunification process.

The court speculated that Jane's mother and grandmother "*may have* contributed to the re-traumatization of the minor child because they are the ones who bring the minor child to these appointments and the minor child seems to be reminded of what has happened." The court further surmised that their "behavior...in *potentially* discussing [Jane's father] and his abuse of the minor child around the minor child and *potentially* reminding her of the abuse is just as abusive to the minor child as what [her father] has done."

In the same order, the court observed that Jane's mother was "hard for the court to understand" and that she "has some mental health issues that need to be addressed and anxiety that is serious in nature; these issues are at least in part related to the stress of this situation [...]." Because of these issues, the court found that her actions in frustrating the father's efforts in the reunification process were not "willful" and did not hold her in contempt. The court then appointed a reunification therapist to conduct reunification therapy and a parenting coordinator to manage the reunification process. Setting target dates for when reunification therapy and supervised visits were to occur, the court made reunification of the minor child with her father the paramount goal despite the lack of evidence to show Jane was no longer at risk of sexual abuse, or that she had healed from the trauma of her experience as a very young child.

Reunification therapy in family courts

As children's attorneys, our office has represented more than seventeen children ordered to reunification therapy where there was a history of the child rejecting contact with a parent or resisting extended periods of visitation. Some of these cases have involved allegations or a history of family violence. Often, the parent accused of abuse has claimed that the accusing parent has alienated the child by coaching the child to fabricate a claim of abuse. For judges who are obligated to rely only on the evidence that is presented in court—where one or both parents may not be represented by counsel and the child has no advocate– identifying the reasons why a child is refusing contact with a parent is extremely challenging. As researchers in the field have noted, too often in divorce situations, all children resisting visits with a parent are improperly labeled alienated, despite the multiplicity of potential reasons for their rejection of the parent (Kelly & Johnston, 2001; Meier, 2003). In 2001, Kelly and Johnston warned that allegations of parental alienation had become "a fashionable legal strategy in numerous divorce cases in which children are resisting contact with a parent, without due regard for possible historic reasons for such resistance within the marital home nor for the children's relationship with both parents" (p. 250). At The Child's Advocate, our experience supports the research that children reject parental contact for a range of different reasons: abuse, exposure to domestic violence, prior periods of abandonment, difficulties with a step parent, a greater affinity between the child and custodial parent predating the divorce, severe denigration of the rejected parent by the custodial parent, or the rejected parent's inability to accept a child's mental illness, disability or sexual orientation.

It is twenty years since Kelly and Johnston warned about the weaponization of claims of parental alienation in family court. Now, such claims are made with ever increasing frequency in custody cases in the U.S. and world-wide, and there is a lucrative and burgeoning industry of "expert" witnesses primed to testify on the issue. Proponents of alienation theories agree, however, that if the child has suffered abuse by the rejected parent, and therefore has a legitimate reason for being estranged from the parent (see Johnston & Kelly for definitions of estrangement vs. alienation), the cause of the child's disaffection should not be attributed to "parental alienation." (Johnston, 2001; Warshak, 2020). For judges with a high volume of cases and a limited amount of court time, reunification therapy holds out the promise of a solution, particularly for those cases designated as "high conflict." Such cases consume a disproportionate share of the court's time and often involve allegations of domestic violence, child maltreatment or parental alienation. Unfortunately, however, when courts do not distinguish between cases involving a high level of conflict versus cases involving legitimate reasons for the child's rejection of a parent, reunification therapy becomes the catch-all remedy to the detriment of some children.

The American Psychological Association does not recognize reunification therapy as an evidence-based treatment, and has not established a set of guidelines, protocols, or best practices for how reunification therapy should be conducted as an evidence-informed practice (Kleinman, 2017; Reitman, 2012). Currently, individual reunification therapists have wide discretion as to how to carry out this form of "therapy." As a child's attorney, I have had multiple clients forced to attend reunification therapy which was then conducted without consideration of trauma-informed principles, particularly in cases where there was evidence of physical, emotional or sexual abuse by the rejected parent.

Importantly, "reunification" or "reparation" therapy ordered in private custody disputes is different from the reunification efforts ordered in juvenile court. In the latter, the state is mandated to attempt to reunify the parent (s) with the child if there has been no termination of parental rights. However, after an adjudication of abuse or neglect in juvenile court, parents who wish to reunify with their children are required to accept responsibility for their neglectful or abusive behavior, and acknowledge the harm suffered by the child (Kleinman, 2017). By contrast, based on the reports of our child clients ordered to reunification therapy while being represented by attorneys with The Child's Advocate—the rejected parent rarely admits or accepts responsibility for past emotional, physical, or sexual abuse or inappropriate parenting. While most reunification therapists do include a phase where the rejected parent is encouraged to acknowledge the child's feelings, our clients usually report their concerns are minimized and they are discouraged from focusing on the past. Such invalidation of children's reasonable complaints significantly undermines a child's trust in her feelings and perceptions and can lead to significant psychological harm. (Lubit, 2019).

Jane's experience of reunification therapy

During an eighteen-month period, Jane attended twelve sessions of reunification therapy and nine supervised community visits with her father. After the ninth visit, Jane's new therapist recommended that supervised visits cease because of the harmful effect they were having on the child's mental health. A few months later, the team discontinued reunification therapy for the same reason. Nonetheless, two years later, Jane's father filed a motion requesting a resumption of reunification therapy, this time asking for a different reunification therapist. He made the sweeping claim, subsequently found to be baseless, that Jane's mother intentionally "interfered in the reunification therapy process by pressuring the minor child when others are not around" and that she "has interfered with him having a relationship with the minor child since her birth and does everything in her power to ensure [he] never sees the child." A month later, Jane's mother filed a motion asking the court to appoint an attorney for her daughter so that Jane could have her "voice" heard by the court and the judge could receive "specialized evidence" about Jane's mental health needs. The court appointed The Child's Advocate, a project of Legal Aid of North Carolina, to represent Jane. A different judge was now presiding over Jane's case.

Representing Jane in family court

After being appointed to represent Jane, I talked with her therapist to learn more about her mental health, something I always do in cases involving a history or allegations of family violence. Jane's therapist, a licensed clinical social worker affiliated with a local university, had extensive expertise in treating sexually abused children. In addition to her clinical practice, she had worked for the county's mental health system assessing parents whose children had been removed because of abuse or neglect, and who were seeking to reunite with their children. I learned from her that Jane was diagnosed with Post Traumatic Stress Disorder (PTSD) at the age of seven and had consistently endorsed sexual abuse and other forms of maltreatment by her father. The reunification process, especially the supervised visits, had greatly exacerbated Jane's PTSD symptoms. When this therapist first began treating her at age nine, the child was experiencing terrifying nightmares focused on her father, she could not sleep in her own bed at night, she had difficulty focusing on her schoolwork and interacting with her peers and was fearful of being alone. In addition, Jane was often sick with allergies and suffered from chronic asthma that was greatly exacerbated by contact with her father. According to her therapist, Jane was a very dutiful child, who had been admonished by her mother to be polite to her father during the supervised visits and reunification sessions. During the two years that followed the termination of reunification, Jane flourished. Her PTSD symptoms were greatly reduced, and the severity of her asthma substantially diminished. Shortly before my appointment as Jane's attorney, the therapist had to tell Jane that her father had petitioned the court to start reunification therapy again. Upon hearing the unwelcome news, the child was tearful and frustrated, venting her anger at her mother and grandmother.

My first meeting with Jane was at her therapist's office. I found my client to be friendly, polite, serious and articulate, with clear ideas about what she wanted to see happen. She was eager to explain to the judge directly why she did not want to attend reunification therapy with her father. In a study of children's participation in decision- making about custody matters, children who had been the subject of protracted, contentious custody disputes were more likely to want to speak directly to the person making the decision (Cashmore & Parkinson, 2007). I explained to Jane that family court judges usually order reunification therapy when a child is refusing contact with a parent, but I was hopeful in her case that the judge would listen carefully to the evidence of how the earlier attempts at reunification had affected her. As I always do with my clients, I emphasized that I could not guarantee an outcome, that her wishes would be one factor among many considered by the judge, but that I would advocate for what she wanted to the best of my ability. Jane seemed relieved at the prospect of having someone who was prepared to bring *her* perspective and *her* experience to the attention of the court.

Jane and I met two more times so I could get to know her better and hear whatever she wanted to share regarding the reasons why she did not want contact with her father. During our meetings, we also discussed her desire to speak directly with the judge. I explained to Jane that the reunification therapist, the visitation supervisor and Jane's own therapist would testify. By asking questions of these witnesses, offering Jane's records into evidence, and advocating for what Jane wanted, I would be able to bring her perspective, concerns and wishes to the court's attention without her having to testify. We agreed she would let me make the final decision as to whether her testimony was necessary to achieve the outcome she desired. A few days prior to trial, we visited the courthouse together so Jane would be familiar with the court environment in the event she needed to speak with the judge. A discussion of the many jurisdictional differences regarding children's access to counsel in family courts across the U.S., as well as how courts may hear and consider the "child's voice", is beyond the scope of this article.

Evidence considered by the court

On the day of trial, the court heard testimony from the supervisor, the reunification therapist, Jane's individual therapist, her parents, and her grandmother. The judge received records of the supervised visits, progress notes from reunification therapy, Jane's psychiatric records and her school report cards. In addition, the court reviewed two pieces of evidence that portrayed starkly contrasting images of Jane's relationship with her father: one was a photo of a smiling Jane and her father posing together for a photo during a supervised community visit; the second was a drawing Jane had done at school a few weeks after the *first* supervised visit had taken place. It showed a terrified little girl begging a female superhero to "save me from my dad" with the word "safe" written beside the image of the superhero.

The supervisor testifies about Jane's visits with her father

The visitation supervisor, a licensed clinical social worker with more than a decade of experience supervising visits, was recommended by the parenting coordinator. Based on handwritten notes taken at the time of the visits, the supervisor had produced a detailed report for each of the nine visits. Each report had a section detailing the activities engaged in by Jane and her father, and sections for the supervisor's observations of Jane's behavior. According to the supervisor's testimony, during the first six visits, Jane engaged very positively with her father, chatted with him, had a photo taken with him, was "giggling and laughing", and looked as though she was really enjoying their interactions. Referring to what she characterized as a sudden shift in Jane's attitude during the last three visits, the supervisor emphasized the changes in Jane's demeanor and affect when her mother would arrive to pick her up at the end of the visits. According to the supervisor, these changes would include Jane abruptly withdrawing from her father. She further testified that after the sixth visit, Jane began complaining that nobody listens to her feelings, that the adults in her life were telling her what to do, and that she wanted the visits to end. The supervisor attributed Jane's withdrawal from her father to the fact that she was "conflicted" in her loyalties to her parents. Consistent with the rules of evidence which do not permit witnesses to testify to what is inside another person's head—i.e., their actual thoughts and feelings–the court sustained repeated objections (made by the mother's counsel and the child's attorney) to the supervisor's attempts to testify to how Jane was feeling and what she was actually thinking during the visits with her father. On cross examination, the supervisor had to admit that *nothing* in her reports or handwritten notes–the latter written at the time of the visits–indicated that Jane's withdrawal from her father become more pronounced when her mother arrived. In fact, she conceded that during many of the visits, Jane was very withdrawn *prior to* her mother's arrival, wanting little to do with the father. She also had to acknowledge that neither her reports nor her notes said anything about Jane's affect and facial expression changing when her mother appeared. The dichotomy between the supervisor's contemporaneous notes versus her recollection of the visits three years later suggests that it was the supervisor's bias that caused her to attribute Jane's withdrawal to the mother's influence rather than to Jane's actual experience of forced visits with a parent who had sexually abused her.

Testimony by the reunification therapist

The reunification therapist conducted a total of fourteen sessions of reunification therapy, twelve of them involving Jane: one with her therapist, some with Jane and each parent, and others with Jane and both parents together. The reunification therapist had email or telephone contact with the parenting coordinator, the two therapists who treated Jane during the reunification process, and Jane's parents. Like the visitation supervisor, the reunification therapist testified to a significant change in Jane's attitude toward her father, a change that the reunification team could not explain. According to the reunification therapist, it was not until the twelfth session that Jane herself made her first "really forceful" statement that she wanted reunification to stop. The reunification therapist conceded, however, that well before the twelfth session, Jane's therapist and mother had informed her that the child was unable to sleep in her own bed, was having frequent nightmares, and was experiencing fear, anger, and a level of anxiety that necessitated medication being prescribed by her psychiatrist. At trial, the reunification therapist agreed that several months before the reunification process was terminated, Jane was literally "begging" for contact to stop. Ultimately, the breaking point appeared to be a session in which the father stated that his long-term goals were to "hug and kiss" his daughter, shortly after Jane clearly stated she did not want him to touch her in any way.

Jane's therapist explains to the court why reunification therapy retraumatized the child

Jane was starting her fifth grade in elementary school when her therapist, three months into treatment, recommended ending the reunification process because of the psychological distress it was causing the child. In the therapist's opinion, Jane's PTSD was precipitated by the child's traumatic experience of sexual abuse by her father. Avoidance, a classic symptom of PTSD, caused Jane to resist any form of therapy that reminded her of her father. She noted that after supervised visits and reunification therapy ceased, Jane flourished and there was a marked reduction in her nightmares and other symptoms. Her social interactions with her peers improved, and she was able to engage in a wide variety of activities during her fifth grade in elementary school- by contrast with her third and fourth grades when chronic health problems prevented her from doing so. While she recommended Trauma Focused Cognitive Behavioral Therapy (TF-CBT) for Jane to help desensitize her to the sexual abuse, the therapist testified she could not begin this treatment while there was any possibility the court would order further contact between Jane and her father. If Jane was not treated for the sexual abuse and its sequelae, Jane would be at risk for long term mental health problems including self-harm, sexual promiscuity, and relationship difficulties.

The court's findings

By contrast with the *sudden* shift in Jane's demeanor toward her father that the supervisor and reunification therapist had observed, the findings made by the court paint a far more nuanced picture. Based on a close review of the supervisor's reports, the reunification therapist's progress notes and the testimony of both professionals, the court determined that the child had alternated between reluctance, nervousness and excitement *before* the supervised visits began. As early as the third community visit, Jane declined her father's hugs, would not allow photos to be taken of herself and her father, and asked the supervisor not to leave her alone with him. At the fifth visit, she told the supervisor that she did not want to be at the visits or have any unsupervised contact with him in the future. Before the sixth visit started, she refused to get out of her mother's car and the supervisor had to persuade her to do so. At the seventh, eighth and ninth visits, Jane told the supervisor she was unable to sleep on her own at night, complaining that no-one had asked her for her feelings about these visits. The court found that after the *first* supervised visit, the reunification therapist received reports from the child's therapist that Jane was experiencing anger and fear. Four months later, Jane told the reunification therapist that she was having nightmares, she worried about the visits while she was at school, and she felt "forced" to participate in the visits. Jane revealed that she was not rude to her father during the visits or during reunification therapy because her mother had warned her to be "polite and respectful." On more than one occasion, Jane referred to "what happened" when she was four and that her feelings were not listened to. The court noted that Jane repeatedly rebuffed her father's hugs during supervised visits.

Among the court's detailed findings were the following: early in the reunification process, Jane's psychiatrist and therapist both diagnosed her with PTSD. During the attempted reunification, Jane and her mother reported the following: fear, crying, emotional outbursts, yelling at her mother, inability to sleep in her own bed, stress-related asthma, anxiety about contact with her father, and continuing nightmares. Jane told her psychiatrist the visits were "against her will", that "she has been trying to be nice to Dad because she is afraid of him, but others have the impression that things are going well." After her first supervised visit, Jane told her psychiatrist about struggling to breathe due to an asthma attack. After Jane had been going through the reunification process for a year, Jane's psychiatrist had to prescribe Lexapro to treat her anxiety. The court noted that six days before the hearing on the father's request to resume reunification therapy, Jane's pediatrician determined she was breathing at just 55% capacity due to stress-induced asthma. Notably, neither Jane's psychiatrist nor her pediatrician—both of whom wrote letters regarding the detrimental impact of forced contact on Jane's health—were a part of the reunification team.

The court denies the father's request to resume reunification

Based on the detrimental effect that reunification was having on Jane, and her therapist's testimony that the possibility of future contact with her father precluded her from engaging in TF-CBT, the judge ruled that a resumption of reunification was not in Jane's best interests.

Termination of the father's parental rights

Six months after entry of the order in family court, Jane's mother filed a petition in juvenile court asking the court to terminate the father's parental rights. The petition was not challenged by him. The juvenile court, after hearing evidence, entered an order terminating his rights, and adopted many of the findings made by the family court judge. The juvenile court judge found by clear and convincing evidence that Jane's "father's involvement in his daughter's life, and his actions, have caused his daughter severe physical and emotional consequences", that he and Jane had an "extremely unhealthy bond," and that "he fails to admit ... that he sexually abused the child." Finally, the judge found that since being informed that reunification therapy would not resume, Jane's "mental health has improved drastically" and "she has continued to express to her therapist she wants her father's rights terminated... and wants the security of knowing she will not be forced to see her father again."

Courts should not order reunification therapy for a child who has been sexually abused

In private custody disputes in family court, cases involving allegations of child sexual abuse are rarely black and white but fall somewhere in the gray area (Hewitt, 2008). Sadly, when Jane was four years old and the court conducted the first hearing on custody, Jane's case was not in a gray zone. Based on the testimony of the CPS supervisor and Jane's treating therapist, the court had made a clear finding that Jane had been sexually abused by her father. Unfortunately, with the passage of time, a second report made to CPS at a time when there was no possibility her father could have abused her, the father's allegations of parental alienation, and the court's conjecture that Jane's mother and grandmother may have re-traumatized Jane, the focus changed to maximizing the father's opportunity to reunify with his daughter. It was not until Jane's new therapist, with expertise in child sexual abuse, presented the court with uncontroverted evidence of the harm that the reunification process was doing to Jane that the court found that a relationship with her father was not in her best interests. By then, Jane was twelve years old. The belief (entrenched in family court) that it is always in a child's best interests to have a relationship with both parents had led the first court to inappropriately order contact between Jane with her father despite his failure to acknowledge or address his harmful conduct in any way (Champion et al., 2020).

By contrast with "reunification therapy" as practiced in family court, there exists an evidence-based, trauma-informed clinical model that professionals seeking to reunify a child with a parent who has sexually offended should follow (Tabachnik & Pollard, 2016). Critical to the likelihood of success are five key steps: a) treatment of the offender, victim, and family by therapists with expertise in child sexual abuse; b) assessment of the readiness of the offender and the child to reunify; c) the offending parent's acceptance of responsibility for the abuse; d) supervised visits in a clinical setting and in the community, and e) ongoing supervision for at least a year. (Gilligan & Bumby, 2005; Price, 2004). Unfortunately, the reunification process experienced by Jane fell far short of the model described above. Because Jane's father continued to deny that he ever sexually abused his daughter and blamed the mother and grandmother for coaching the child, he was never required to be treated by a therapist with expertise in treating offending parents. Likewise, the individual therapist who treated Jane during the first fifteen months of the reunification process was not required to have, and to this writer's knowledge did not have, specialized training in child sexual abuse. Moreover, the court never ordered an assessment of whether Jane was ready for reunification by a professional with expertise in child sexual abuse. Price highlights the importance of such an assessment taking place:

> It is essential that those involved in making this assessment fully understand the nuances of complex developmental, emotional, psychological, cognitive, and trauma-related factors involved. For this reason, a clinician who has been trained specifically in working with children who have experienced sexual abuse should direct the assessment.

Ironically, Jane's mother was the only member of the family, who, during the attempted reunification process, received treatment delivered by providers with expertise in child sexual abuse. CPS provided the mother with group and individual therapeutic services specifically tailored to non-offending parents. As discussed later in this article, supervised visitation was conducted by a supervisor who did not implement protocols recommended for visits involving sexually abused children (Hewitt, 2008). Ultimately, the lack of trauma-informed practices delivered by providers with the necessary expertise resulted in Jane being re-traumatized over an eighteen- month period through forced contact with her father.

Implicit bias may cause professionals to mistakenly assume parental alienation

As I prepared for the hearing, I contacted the supervisor to speak with her about my client's participation in supervised visits. According to her, the case was clearly about "parental alienation." Unfortunately, her endorsement of parental alienation, which the court later deemed to be baseless, served to buttress the claims that the father's attorneys had been making throughout the litigation. Prior to trial, the father's attorney referred to Jane as the victim of "long-standing alienation," clearly expecting the supervisor's testimony to confirm this. Several writers have written of family courts' over-reliance on "neutral" professionals in custody determinations (Lubit, 2019: Meier, 2003). Basing his analysis on a sample of child custody evaluations, Lubit illustrates the circular logic employed by some child custody evaluators who, by analyzing the facts of the custody cases through the lens of parental alienation, proceed to identify parental alienation as the *cause* of the child's resistance to contact with a parent. Likewise, other researchers have cautioned against excessive reliance on putatively "neutral" professionals such as GALs, reunification therapists, custody evaluators, and parenting coordinators in cases involving family violence. A lack of specialized training in domestic violence and child abuse often results in these "neutral" professionals inserting their own personal values and assumptions and failing to recognize the legitimate reasons a child may have for rejecting a parent (Ducote, 2002; Meier,

2003; Milchman, 2017). Similarly, other researchers have warned of the critical need to screen for family violence and other factors before a determination of parental alienation is made. (Saunders & Faller, 2016).

Ultimately, the judge rebuffed the claim that alienation was the cause of the failed attempt to reunify Jane and her father and found there was "insufficient credible evidence to suggest the mother had anything to do with the child not wanting to participate in reunification therapy or did anything to lead to the child's distress over reunification therapy." As Milchman (2017) has noted, judicial oversight can be a critical check against implicit bias by court-appointed professionals. After delivering her decision and stating the findings she wanted included in the order, the judge specifically instructed the attorneys not to "deflect causality" to Jane's mother for the child's distress over the attempted reunification with her father.

An early email from Jane's individual therapist to the reunification team provides further evidence that the narrative of parental alienation was false. Written some months after reunification therapy began, but before Jane began supervised visits, her individual therapist emailed the reunification team for guidance, stating:

> (Mom) has told (Jane) that she is working hard to have a better future with (Dad), but when (Mom) attempted to state positive things about (Dad), (Jane) said (Mom) was trying to put words in (Jane's) mouth, and she does not think (Dad) is positive. (Jane) has also expressed anger at her mom for "making her" see her (Dad), [...].

The supervisor's bias affected how she supervised Jane's visits with her father

As a professional required to maintain an unbiased environment (Supervised Visitation Network, 2006), the supervisor failed to maintain a neutral role. Nor did she follow recommended protocols for supervised visits where child sexual abuse is a concern (Hewitt, 2008). For example, she did not have the father agree in advance to specific rules regarding appropriate physical contact. When questioned about the father's repeated requests for hugs from his daughter, and his failure to observe the child's boundaries, the supervisor defended him at trial, saying, "he didn't do it perfectly… none of us do." Although the supervisor told the father he needed to ask his child for permission before hugging her, she allowed him to *repeatedly* ask Jane for hugs despite the child rebuffing him. As one report states: "Jane allowed her father to tie her shoes, gather her belongings and then gave him *the hug he had wanted most of the afternoon*." According to the supervisor, the father asking his daughter for hugs was "a natural way of building a relationship with a child"-notwithstanding her knowledge of the court's prior finding that Jane had been sexually abused.

In Jane's case, the supervisor's opinion that the mother was to blame for the child's rejection of her father proved to be an unfounded hunch—and one she was not allowed to speculate about at trial. However, under different circumstances, as one of the two "neutral" professionals who had the opportunity to directly observe Jane's interactions with her father, the supervisor's testimony that Jane had six successful visits with her father could have led the court to give the father another opportunity to reunify. As other researchers have cautioned, a child's behavior during observation in a physically safe environment is not a valid indication of whether the child feels comfortable with the parent or has been victimized in the past (Bancroft & Silverman, 2002; Faller et al., 1991). In this case, cross-examination by competent attorneys, and a conscientious, trauma-informed judge prevented the supervisor's clear alignment with the father from adversely influencing the outcome.

A child needs an attorney in cases involving allegations of child abuse or domestic violence

Our adversarial judicial system is based on the premise that the parties to a dispute, through counsel, present evidence supporting their respective positions. Once that evidence is subjected to cross-examination, the fact finder is supposed to be able to resolve the conflicting accounts and arrive at the truth. The reality of family court is very different. Cases like Jane's where the parties *and the child* are all represented by competent counsel are the exception. In the vast majority of child custody cases in North Carolina, the child has neither an attorney nor a lay advocate. In many cases, neither parent has an attorney; in others, one parent is represented by counsel and the other is not. In the courts where attorneys from The Child's Advocate are appointed, over-worked and under-resourced judges struggle to manage over-crowded dockets. Apart from mandatory mediation for the litigants, there are *no* state-funded resources available for the child or parents. If the case goes to trial, the court must depend on the parties to present the critical evidence upon which the court must base its decision. Even when both parents are represented—and the playing field is leveled in theory—custody decisions are greatly affected by the relative competency of the attorneys, the training and experience of the judges, the skills (and bias) of the family court professionals who testify, and most importantly, by the evidence that the court receives.

The difficulty of presenting evidence of child abuse in family court

In family court, it is notoriously difficult to prove that child sexual abuse has occurred. Frequently, there is no physical evidence of abuse, myths about child sexual abuse are exploited by defense counsel, and the victim is often a child too young or too vulnerable to testify. Presenting evidence of child sexual abuse requires an attorney with training in this area, who can issue and *enforce* subpoenas for medical and mental health providers, and who can ensure that the court receives all relevant records (CPS, psychiatric, psychological and medical, etc.). The fees for retaining counsel to bring such a case to trial are often prohibitive, not to mention the costs of depositions, psychological evaluations, expert testimony, etc. If the accused parent has raised the charge of parental alienation, the likelihood that the court will credit an allegation of child sexual abuse is significantly diminished. The national study conducted by Meier (2020) tracks how courts have ruled in cases involving claims of child abuse and charges of parental alienation. The following statistics from Meier's study underscore the extraordinary difficulty of proving child sexual abuse: out of two hundred cases involving an allegation of child sexual abuse, the court credited the claim—i.e., believed that child sexual abuse had occurred– in just twenty-nine of those cases. In the fifty cases where the father counter-charged with a claim of parental alienation, only *one* claim of child sexual abuse was credited by the court. Given that outside research by impartial researchers indicates that claims of child sexual abuse are valid between 50%–72% of the time (Faller, 1998), the results of Meier's national study highlight the need for systemic changes to ensure that family courts are protecting children from sexual abuse by a parent.

Why a child needs an attorney to ensure that court receives the evidence it needs

The Child's Advocate, a project of Legal Aid of North Carolina, offers judges in Wake, Durham, Orange and Chatham counties the opportunity to appoint attorneys–from our office and the private family law bar–to represent children in contentious custody cases involving allegations of domestic violence, child abuse, maltreatment, etc. The American Bar Association recognizes two distinct types of attorneys for children—a child's attorney and a best interests attorney (American Bar Association Section of Family Law Standards of Practice for Lawyers Representing Children in Custody Cases, 2003). Our office, however, only accepts appointments to serve as a child's attorney, i.e., where we advocate for our clients' expressed interests and objectives. We favor this model of representation because our goal is to bring the *child*'s perspective to the table, not *our assessment* of what is in the child's best interests. When a child is resisting contact with a parent, the other court-appointed professionals—reunification therapists, parenting coordinators, GALs, best-interests attorneys, custody evaluators—base their recommendations on *their* assessment of what is in the child's best interests. Without a child's attorney, the court does not hear from any witness whose exclusive duty is to bring the child's experience, perspective and wishes to the forefront. Moreover, cross examination of the court-appointed professionals whose implicit biases may influence their testimony is a legal check that protects children (Milchman, 2017). In Jane's case, the child was twelve before the court heard any evidence of Jane's perspective on having a relationship with her father—one that was dramatically different from the perceptions of the court-appointed professionals involved. Ultimately, it was only through the appointment of an attorney for Jane, a close collaboration between that attorney and Jane's therapist, the presentation of detailed documentary evidence, and cross-examination of witnesses by attorneys for both Jane and her mother, that the court received the critical testimony of how forced reunification had re-traumatized Jane.

Jane's experience of the court-ordered process is a text-book example of the importance of an advocate who will listen to the child's voice, credit what the child is saying, *and* present the evidence that supports the child's perspective. As researchers in the UK have shown through their study of children from divorced families, "children are not only relevant and competent witnesses to the process of their parents' divorce, they are also the most reliable witnesses of their own experience" (Butler et al., 2002). Similarly, the Speaking for Themselves (SFT) project underscores the value of crediting what children have to say. This project, undertaken in Calgary, Canada, combined a child's attorney with a trauma therapist for children caught in contentious custody disputes involving domestic violence. (Fotheringham et al., 2013). Based on the belief that children in custody disputes involving family violence are entitled to a voice in decisions that affect their lives, children received therapeutic counseling from a trauma therapist and legal representation by an attorney to ensure that their needs, rights and views were considered by judges making decisions regarding custody and access. In 89% of SFT cases, both children and therapists agreed on what the best outcome would be. Over eighty percent of the actual outcomes reflected children's opinions of what they wanted to have happen. These statistics show that in custody cases involving family violence, what children wanted—the custodial/access arrangement they favored—most often coincided with what the therapist and the court determined to be in their best interests.

Judge Karen Adams, with decades of experience in both juvenile and family court in Tucson, Arizona, is clear about the need for a child's attorney in almost every child custody case. (Adams, 2007). While juvenile court is philosophically welcoming to the child's attorney-who is regarded as an integral part of the juvenile proceeding—in family court, by contrast, "children must fight to be heard in family law cases, where often decisions are made for and about them without the judge knowing their position." After she began appointing *pro bono* attorneys for children in cases with a high level of conflict, substance abuse, family violence, or mental health issues, Judge Adams concluded that a "child's attorney" as defined by the ABA standards was the most effective way for the court to receive information about the child's perspective, and thereby "fill the very large gap between what is presented in court and what the judge really needs to know." Adams made a point of ensuring that appointed attorneys understood their role and did not act as best interests' attorneys.

As children's attorneys, we do not claim to be immune from bias. However, by continually reminding ourselves of our clients' goals and our duty to advocate for those goals, we are less likely to allow our own personal values and cultural assumptions to influence our advocacy. In order to understand our clients, many of whom have endured the turmoil of years of custody litigation, emotional, physical or sexual abuse, a parent's mental illness or substance abuse, harsh parenting, or ongoing severe denigration of one parent by the other, we provide trauma-informed legal representation. We receive ongoing training on family violence, the effects of trauma on children and adults, the consequences of exposure to domestic violence. We also keep abreast of the current research on parental alienation.

What Jane wrote in her journal during the coerced contact with her father

If I had needed any assurance that what Jane told me was not the product of her mother's influence, all I needed to do was look at the private journal kept by Jane while reunification was being attempted. When the nine-year old girl would awaken screaming from her sleep because of nightmares about her father, she could not go to her mother for comfort because any discussion about her father was prohibited. What follows is a selection of Jane's entries, the first entry written five days before her first supervised visit, and the last entry made after a reunification session with her father some five months later. A few entries were made in the early hours of the morning. Jane addresses an unknown reader:

> Dear?
>
> people don't listen to me. please help me because i need my life to be better. please. help.
>
> 8/17/15, 1 a.m. my nightmare was about how daddy's minions trapped me in the night and daddy killed (my doll) and i tried to get her back but i couldn't and I will always be crying

8/18/15, 4 a.m. my nightmare was about how daddy locked me in a closet and when I got out all of my stuffed animals were hurt.

9/13/15 (the supervisor) e- mailed my mom and asked where i want to go next with my dad so i told my mommy that I don't want to go anywhere with him. i feel scared. question is why do i have to be with someone i am scared of.

i said no to a hug I don't want to be there

11/14/15: i have went to 2 visits it was very stressful.

i'm not lying about dad doing stuff to me.

11/15/15 i need a big break from seeing all these and from seeing my dad. its making me sick i want to be a normal kid

12/1/15: i feel like people are thinking that I'm lying about dad doing stuff to me. but i'm not. and that (supervisor)is lying about my visits. and I do tell her that I feel uncomfortable. that its too much stress on a 9 year old. can't they wait until i am a teenager so that I can handle the stress better?

why do people put this much pressure. don't they care about me. why do they pressure me. (the supervisor) makes me be nice. they listen to my dad more than me. i don't like my dad!!

(the supervisor) says to me that she is in charge and that I do whatever she says.

is there rules. can i leave when i want to leave because (the supervisor) wouldn't let me.

12/12/15: I said the reason that (I was) playing nice was because I don't want to get into trouble (my mother) told me to be polite and makes me go

12/13/15 (my grandmother) wants me to sleep in my own bed. because i have a lot of nightmares i think that my dad is going to capture me but when i sleep with someone they protect me.

12/15/15: At my visit I said I hate my dad. I don't want to be with my dad. I am mad!!

I was hitting my dad in my dream but accidentally kicked my grandma instead

Two years later

Jane is now fifteen years old and living with her mother and grandparents in another state. It is clear from my interactions with Jane over zoom that she is blossoming. She is animated and expressive and happy as she tells me about her about her new life. Jane shared with me that during the forced reunification process she frequently engaged in stress-eating to help her deal with the anxiety—so much so that she weighed one hundred and seventy-six pounds at the height of the reunification efforts. Soon after learning her father's rights had been terminated, Jane felt motivated to eat healthy food and to work out regularly. She has lost forty pounds since the reunification process ended. Her asthma has greatly improved, and when we last spoke Jane had not needed to use an inhaler in several months. Jane credits the courts' decision to deny reunification therapy and to terminate her father's rights with "giving [her] back [her] life". I invited Jane and her mother to share any suggestions they wanted to make so other children would not be subjected to coerced contact with an offending parent.

Recommendations (based on Jane's case and other cases handled by The Child's Advocate)

In cases involving child abuse or exposure to domestic violence: a) courts should appoint a child's attorney so that the court receives evidence of the child's actual experience. Jane believes that children should have their own advocate so they have a better understanding of what is happening in court, are included in the conversation, and the focus is on the child instead of the adults; b) courts should not send children to reunification therapy without having the child assessed by an independent mental health professional with expertise in the particular area of concern (e.g. child sexual abuse); c) if reunification is still ordered, then it should be delivered by professionals with expertise in the area of concern. Jane's mother describes the professionals involved in Jane's case as attempting to navigate "unchartered territory."

A child's individual therapist should be independent of the reunification process. Jane told me that the first therapist who treated her during reunification kept pressuring her to have contact with her father, discouraged her from saying anything "bad" about him, and was suspicious that Jane was being influenced by others. Jane said it felt like her therapist was working on behalf of her father. By her own report, this experience left her feeling more "unstable."

Judges and all court-appointed professionals should have to meet *stringent*, uniform requirements for ongoing and specialized training in child abuse, domestic violence and trauma. The need for stringent requirements is illustrated by the fact that the visitation supervisor testified to having attended multiple trainings in trauma and child abuse matters, but her actual supervision did not reflect trauma-informed principles. Protective parents in custody cases involving allegations of child abuse and domestic violence should have access to supportive services. Jane's mother described how she was "silently screaming" as she watched her daughter suffer throughout the reunification process. The therapeutic services for non-offending parents that she received from CPS were critical to maintaining her sanity.

Acknowledgments

I am indebted to Jane and her mother for permitting me to share Jane's story. I thank my colleagues at Legal Aid of NC who have given me valuable feedback and advice on this article. I am grateful to attorneys at The Child's Advocate and *pro bono* attorneys from the family law bar who, every day, bring the child's voice to the table in contentious custody disputes. Finally, I owe a debt of gratitude to Sally Scherer, J.D., for her vision in founding The Child's Advocate in 2009.

Disclosure of interest

Author has no conflict of interest to disclose. The authors alone are responsible for the content and writing of the paper.

Ethical standards and informed consent

This article is a retrospective analysis of a custody case involving reunification. Jane and her mother have given informed consent to the use of Jane's story. No experimentation was involved.

References

Adams, K. S. (2007). Make Room at Counsel Table for the Child's Attorney. *Family Advocate*. (reprinted in GPSolo, the ABA magazine for the General Practice, Solo and Small Firm Division, "Best of ABA Sections" Issue, September 2009).

American Bar Association Section of Family Law Standards of Practice for Lawyers Representing Children in Custody Cases. (2003) *37* Fam. L.Q. 129.

Bancroft, L. R., & Silverman, J. G. (2002). *The batterer as parent: Addressing the impact of domestic violence on family dynamics*. Sage.

Butler, I., Scanlan, L., Robinson, M., Douglas, G., & Murch, M. (2002). Children's involvement in their parents' divorce: Implications for practice. *Children & Society*, *16*(2), 89–102. https://doi.org/10.1002/chi.702

Cashmore, J., & Parkinson, P. (2007). What responsibility do courts have to hear children's voices. *International Journal of Children's Rights*, *15*, 43–60.

Champion, K. M., et al. (2020). Intimate partner violence and family court. In R. Geffner. (Ed.), *Handbook of interpersonal violence across the lifespan*. https://doi.org/10.1007/978-3-319-62122-7_314-1

Dallam, S., & Silberg, J. L. (2016). Recommended treatments for "parental alienation syndrome" (PAS) may cause children foreseeable and lasting psychological harm. *Journal of Child Custody*, *13* (2-3), 134–143. https://doi.org/10.1080/15379418.2016.1219974

Dimidjian, S., & Hollon, S. D. (2010). How would we know if psychotherapy were harmful?*American Psychologist*, *65*(1), 21–33. https://doi.org/10.1037/a0017299

Ducote, R. (2002). Guardians ad litem in private custody litigation: the case for abolition. *Loyola Journal of Public Interest Law, 3*, 106–151.

Faller, K. C. (1998). The Parental Alienation Syndrome: What is it and What Data Support it? *Child Maltreatment, 3*(2), 100–107. https://doi.org/10.1177/1077559598003002005

Faller, K. C., Froning, M., & Lipovsky, J. (1991). The parent-child interview: Its use in evaluating child allegations of sexual abuse by the parent. *American Journal of Orthopsychiatry, 61*(4), 552–557. https://doi.org/10.1037/h0079286

Fidler, B. J., Bala, N., et al. (2012). *Children who resist post-separation parental contact: a differential approach for legal and mental health professionals*. Oxford University Press.

Fotheringham, S., Dunbar, J., & Hensley, D. (2013). Speaking for Themselves: Hope for Children Caught in High Conflict Custody and Access Disputes Involving Domestic Violence. *Journal of Family Violence, 28*(4), 311–324. https://doi.org/10.1007/s10896-013-9511-3

Gilligan, L., Bumby, K. (2005). Key considerations for reunifying adult sex offenders and their families. Retrieved from Center for Sex Offender Management: http://www/csom.org/pubs/familyreunificationdec05.pdf.

Hewitt, S. K. (2008). Therapeutically managing reunification after abuse allegations. *Journal of Child Sexual Abuse, 17*(1), 17–19. https://doi.org/10.1080/10538710701884326

Kelly, J. B., & Johnston, J. R. (2001). The Alienated Child: A Reformulation of Parental Alienation Syndrome. *Family Court Review, 39*(3), 249–266. https://doi.org/10.1111/j.174-1617.2001.tb00609.x

Kleinman, T. (2017). Family court ordered "reunification therapy": junk science in the guise of helping parent/child relationships? *Journal of Child Custody, 14*(4), 295–300. https://doi.org/10.1080/15379418.2017.1413699

Lubit, R. (2019). Valid and invalid ways to assess the reason a child rejects a parent: The continued malignant role of 'parental alienation syndrome. *Journal of Child Custody, 16*(1), 42–66. https://doi.org/10.1080/15379418.2019.1590284

Meier, J. S. (2003). Domestic violence, child custody, and child protection: understanding judicial resistance and imagining the solutions. *American University Journal of Gender Social Policy and Law, 11*(2), 657–730.

Meier, J. S. (2020). U.S. child custody outcomes in cases involving parental alienation and abuse allegations: what do the data show? *Journal of Social Welfare and Family Law, 42*(1), 92–105. https://doi.org/10.1080/09649069.2020.1701941

Mercer, J. (2019). Are intensive parental alienation treatments effective and safe for children and adolescents?*Journal of Child Custody, 16*(1), 67–113. https://doi.org/10.1080/15378418.2018.1557578

Milchman, M. S. (2017). Misogyny in New York custody decisions with parental alienation versus child sexual abuse allegations. *Journal of Child Custody, 14*(4), 234–259. https://doi.org/10.1080/15379418.2017.1416723

Price, D. M. (2004). Rebuilding shattered families: Disclosure, clarification, and reunification of sexual abusers, victims, and their families. *Sexual Addiction & Compulsivity, 11*(4), 187–221.

Reitman, P. (2012). Reunification therapy. https://paulreitman.files.wordpress.com/2012/02/reunification1.pdf

Saunders, D. G., & Faller, K. C. (2016). The need to carefully screen for family violence when parental alienation is claimed. *Michigan Family Law Journal, 46*(6), 7–11.

Silberg, J., & Dallam, S. (2019). Abusers gaining custody in family courts: a case series of over-turned decisions. *Journal of Child Custody, 16*(2), 140–169. https://doi.org/10.1080/15379418.2019.1613204

Supervised Visitation Network. (2006). Supervised Visitation Network. Standards for supervised visitation practice Prepared by: SVN Standards Task Force and the Standards and Guidelines Committee.

Tabachnik, J., & Pollard, P. (2016). *Considering family reconnections and reunification after child sexual abuse: A road map for advocates and service providers*. National Sexual Violence Resource Center.

Warshak, R. A. (2020). When evaluators get it wrong: false positive IDs and parental alienation. *Psychology, Public Policy, and Law*, *26*(1), 54–68. https://doi.org/10.1037/law0000216

Reunification therapies for parental alienation: Tenets, empirical evidence, commonalities, and differences

Jean Mercer

ABSTRACT
Reunification therapies (RTs) for parental alienation are intended to repair relationships between parents and children who have rejected contact with those parents as a result of manipulation by preferred parents. Proponents of intensive (four day to several weeks) RTs have published outcome studies and other reports. This paper examines six intensive RTs that share some basic assumptions: Family Bridges, Family Reflections Reunification Program, High Road to Reunification, Overcoming Barriers Family Camp, Transitioning Families Therapeutic Reunification Model, and Turning Points for Families. Tenets, treatment methods, and outcomes of each program are critiqued. It is concluded that many program tenets are questionable, and that outcome studies are too weakly designed and implemented to provide evidence of the programs' effectiveness. Information about these programs is thus concluded not to be admissible as scientific evidence in the courtroom.

Reunification therapies (RTs; also called reintegration and reconnection therapies) are psychological treatments used when a child of divorced parents resists or refuses contact with one parent. Miller (2022) extends the situation to include lack of a "normal relationship" in the context of regular contact with the parent. In many cases of resistance or refusal, it is argued that parental alienation (PA) is the cause of the child's attitude; this argument posits that some children who resist or refuse contact have been persuaded to do so by the alienating actions of the preferred parent.

RTs are often thought of as especially relevant to PA cases, even though resistance or refusal of contact may result from non-PA causes like previous psychological or physical abuse or situational factors like the presence of a stepparent. One parent's poor parenting skills may bring about repeated events which, while individually nowhere near the level of abuse, nevertheless accumulate distressingly and cause a child's negative attitude.

The present paper describes a series of RTs used in cases where PA is alleged, critiques the assumptions and theories on which each treatment is based, and assesses the empirical evidence for the safety and effectiveness of each treatment for which such evidence is available.

Shared aspects of reunification therapies (RTs)

Although there are RTs that are conducted in office settings, the treatments we will consider here are "intensives" that take from several days to several weeks to perform. These RTs share a number of important factors. The first and probably most significant is the court-ordered prohibition of contact between the child and the preferred parent for at least 90 days, accompanied by reversal of custody so that the child is in the care of the rejected parent. A second critical component is the child's participation in a "workshop" or "camp" lasting from four days to several weeks and intended to soften or eliminate the child's rejection and encourage the building of a good relationship with the formerly rejected parent. Third, intensive RTs require participation by the preferred parent in treatment by a practitioner approved by the RT program, including in some cases the writing of a letter to the child explaining that the preferred parent has acted to "brainwash" the child and now regrets this; the preferred parent is also required to pay much of the substantial costs of the RT program. The present author has seen estimates of $20,000 to $40,000 for a 4-day RT program. In addition, one parent against whom PA is alleged has estimated that four hours per week of supervised visitation with her children will cost $700 for the week, and the parenting coach she must consult charges $500 per hour.) Failure to comply leads to extended prohibition of contact with the child and may result in judicial findings of contempt of court by the preferred parent.

Problematic tenets behind intensive RTs

A theory is a framework that connects observed events with each other and posits a supportable mechanism by which events influence other events. Conceptualizing PA and developing theory has been difficult because of the lack of systematic observation and the continued absence of a protocol for identifying PA cases. Statements about the child behaviors construed as alienation continue to derive primarily from Gardner's (1985) description of his patients. Statements about the alienating behaviors of the preferred parent tend to be based on Baker's (e.g., Baker, 2005) work, in which she invited community adults to describe what they recalled of a parent's behavior. There are no published frequency counts comparing either child or parent behavior to that in cases where PA is not alleged. In addition, discussion of PA continues to describe "brainwashing" as the mechanism by which a preferred parent causes a child to reject the other parent, even though "brainwashing" has long been considered a legal rather than a psychological concept (Reichert et al., 2015) and therefore does not provide a supportable mechanism for understanding PA cases. As a result, there is actually no theory of PA.

There is, however, a PA belief system that depends on a series of shared, but largely questionable, tenets. These *a priori* assumptions underlie intensive RT programs. It is less clear whether they are similarly at work in office-based RTs. Here is a list of tenets shared by intensive RT programs; many of the tenets have been critiqued and rejected elsewhere (Mercer, 2021, 2022; Milchman, 2022):

1. It is possible to accurately identify and measure PA .
2. PA is either binary or quantifiable, so differences between pre- and post-treatment can be ascertained and analyzed.
3. Children need both parents for normal development
4. Children need a male and a female parent.
5. Untreated children in PA cases will experience problems with later relationships, as well as overwhelming guilt for their actions toward the rejected parent.
6. RT corrects problems of emotional development.
7. RTs are psychoeducation rather than psychotherapy.
8. Alienating behavior is family violence.
9. It is harmful to children for their preferences to be considered.
10. PA can be treated effectively only when the child is prohibited from contact with the preferred parent and placed in the custody of the rejected parent.
11. Treatment should focus entirely on the present and future interactions of parent and child, without discussion or explanation of past events.

Some RTs also include these further assumptions:

12. Attachment is an issue in PA.
13. Biological and evolutionary reasons make it unnatural to reject a parent, and even children placed in foster care because of abuse do not reject their parents.

Evaluating effectiveness and safety of intensive RTs

This section of the paper will examine a group of intensive RTs with respect to individual assumptions or theories (beyond the shared assumptions discussed earlier), treatment methods, and evidence of effectiveness and safety. Comments here will draw on earlier work by Mercer (2019) and Trane et al. (2022) as well as considering recent publications stating support of RTs. The RTs being examined will be taken in alphabetical order: Family Bridges, Family Reflections Reunification Program, High Road to Reunification, Overcoming Barriers, Transitioning Families Therapeutic Reunification Model, and Turning Points for Families Family Camp. (Although Trane et al., [2022] included Child Centered Conjoint Therapy [Greenberg et al., 2019] in their review, this program is omitted here because it does not focus specifically on PA cases.)

Family bridges

Tenets

In addition to commitment to the shared tenets discussed earlier, Family Bridges is a program based on the idea that PA results from the child's cognitive distortions fostered by the preferred parent via alienating behaviors. According to Warshak (2010), the problem of PA is parallel to the negative attitudes of internationally abducted children returned to the United States and placed with the non-abducting parent. Warshak noted that the California psychologist Randy Rand developed a treatment program for abducted children, and because the problems were seen as parallel, Family Bridges was developed as a parallel form of treatment incorporating Rand's methods.

Warshak's discussion of cognitive distortions used the term "critical thinking" to describe the children's posited cognitive problems, but no specific critical thinking problems were described except that the children were said to be unaware that someone could manipulate their beliefs. The present author would suggest that any cognitive distortions among children from 9 to 12 years of age might well involve their capacity to use what Piaget (see Wadsworth, 2019) called formal operational thought, a set of cognitive skills that allow the thinker to consider multiple factors as they interact and bring about an outcome. Formal operational thought can vary from one domain to another, and is more readily applied to familiar than to unfamiliar material (Burbules & Linn, 1988). Adult emotions and aspects of marital conflict are probably unfamiliar to children in PA cases, and it is possible that increasing their familiarity with this material could help them to think about their family situation in a more mature way, but Warshak does not seem to have discussed this in print.

Treatment methods

Family Bridges admits children and adolescents who are court-ordered for treatment following recommendations of mental health professionals to the court. The orders include no contact with the preferred parent, usually initially for 90 days. Children may be taken to the treatment venue by youth transportion service workers, according to Warshak (2020) and Barnett et al. (2022). Children are allowed no contact with the preferred parent, but the rejected parent is present and engages in the program. The four-day program itself involves watching videos about the nature of attitudes and persuasion, including a video created by Warshak, entitled "Welcome Back, Pluto". Games, family discussions concentrating on present and future, and treats like shopping and dining out are part of the program. Following the four days, parent and child are to go on a vacation together and then return home to live together. Further "aftercare" sessions are to take place with a therapist approved by the program.

Meanwhile, the preferred parent is to have been involved in treatment with a program-approved therapist. Failure to attend or to satisfy the therapist's criteria may result in the parent being found in contempt of court. In a personal communication, one such parent has reported that she was required to write a letter to the children explaining that she had been the cause of their alienation and stating her regret for this.

Effectiveness

As is the case for other RTs, outcome studies for Family Bridges are limited by the absence of an established method of identifying and measuring PA. Entry into the program depends on a court's decision that PA is present, although Warshak (2019) noted that 15% of the admitted children were not refusing contact with the parent; exactly what criteria led to the court orders is not clear. Post-treatment measures did not depend on court decisions, but on questionnaire responses. According to Warshak (2019), parents completed questionnaires before the workshop, responding to questions about the child's cooperation with the court-ordered parenting schedule; the level of their children's rejection, withdrawal and contempt; the quality of the relationship between parent and child; and the extent to which improvements in the relationship were attributed to the Family Bridges program. Following the program, the rejected parents, the children, and the workshop leaders responded to the questionnaire. It is notable that the preferred parents were not asked to respond to the questionnaires. The questionnaires consisted primarily of 4-point Likert-type response choices, which were inappropriately analyzed with *t*-tests rather than the appropriate nonparametric statistics (see Morris et al., 2017; these authors referred to the inappropriate test choice as quantitative alchemy). The series of *t*-tests in fact increased probability of a Type I error (concluding that there was a greater than chance difference between pretreatment and post-treatment scores when in fact there was not.) As a final point, the lack of an untreated control group or any other standard of comparison leaves it quite unclear whether any pre- and post-treatment differences were in fact caused by the Family Bridges experience.

The considerations just outlined suggest that Warshak was mistaken in his conclusion that Family Bridges has been shown to be an effective treatment.

Potential for harm

Lilienfeld (2007), Dimidjian and Hollon (2010), Linden (2013), and others have discussed the need for attention to potential harmfulness of a psychological treatment. Warshak (2019) noted that about 6% of the children in his outcome study did not develop improve d attitudes toward the rejected parent but remained intransigent. He did not, however, report any measure of harm to family members. Barnett et al. (2022) discussed the distressing experience of a child in the Family Bridges program. There have been no measures of possible long-term harm caused by this or similar RT programs.

Although Family Bridges, like other RTs advocates for child relationships with both parents, published reports do not include any information about the child's later contact with the preferred parent, a matter that is a possible source of harm.

Family reflections reunification program

Tenets

Family Reflections (FRRP; Reay, 2015) Shares with Family Bridges the assumption that a child's rejection of a parent is caused by cognitive distortions fostered by the preferred parent. According to Reay (2015), "Alienated children literally have their critical thinking taken away and are forced to align with the cult leader [parent]....Without exposure to healthy people, these children's actions become increasingly bizarre, including accusing the rejected parent of a host of horrible behaviors that he or she has never done" (p. 3.)

Treatment methods

FRRP combines the techniques of Family Bridges, including "multimedia learning" (Reay, 2015), and those of a camp-like experience comparable to Overcoming Barriers (described later in this section). Children are usually court-ordered into the program, with the order including prohibition of all contact with the preferred parent. Children initially attend FRRP without either parent being present and are later joined by the rejected parent; both parent and child experience psychoeducational and other treatments before meeting. The preferred parent is to receive treatment from a practitioner approved by FRRP.

Effectiveness

Reay (2015) reported outcome studies involving 22 children whose initial level of PA was assessed by looking at child custody reports, rejected parents' reports, court reports, and the failure of previous counseling efforts. (Preferred parents did not provide reports.) Peri- and post-treatment assessments considered children's statements, parents' statements, and staff observations. The outcome study reported that 95% of the children established a relationship with the parent between the second and third days of treatment and maintained the relationship. No details were provided about the nature of the evaluations, nor was any statistical analysis given. Reay concluded that FRRP was an effective treatment for PA and did not note the implications of the absence of any control group and the differences in the nature of the pretreatment and post-treatment assessments.

These considerations suggest that Reay was mistaken in her conclusion that FRRP's effectiveness had been demonstrated.

Potential harms

No statements about potential harms associated with FRRP have been published.

High road to reunification

N.B. Other RTs discussed in this paper have been discussed by their proponents in peer-reviewed professional journals. This is not true of High Road to Reunification, which has been described in two self-published books and a document intended for parents whose children are attending the treatment (Conscious Co-Parenting Institute, n.d.) Because High Road is still recommended in some PA cases and on an Internet site (conscious-coparenting.com), it seems worthwhile to consider the treatment here.

Tenets

Childress (2015, 2018) has been the major advocate of High Road to Reunification, which he says was actually created by his colleague, the life coach Dorcy Pruter. In addition to the shared assumptions mentioned earlier in this paper, Childress uses aspects of attachment theory in his explanation of PA. He argues that all children are attached to both their parents, and that when a child resists or refuses contact with a parent, the child does so because his or her attachment system has been "suppressed" by the actions of the preferred parent. Childress does not explain how the attachment system could be suppressed or relate this suppression to the exploratory or other systems posited by Bowlby (Bretherton, 1992). He does, however, suggest that High Road to Reunification rapidly removes the suppression of the attachment system and allows the child to feel attached to the parent once more. These references to attachment ignore the fact that proximity-seeking attachment behavior in toddlers is a different matter from the internal working model of social relations (see Pietromonaco & Barrett, 2000), derived from attachment and other experiences, that governs social interactions in older children, adolescents, and adults.

References to attachment theory are often taken as powerful arguments in legal proceedings, as the evidence for attachment is presumed to be derived from biological and evolutionary information. Mistaken applications of attachment theory like those suggested by Childress should be challenged (see Garber et al., 2021).

Treatment methods

High Road to Reunification depends on unique methods of identifying PA (Childress, 2015, 2018) and treatment methods that resemble Family Bridges and other RTs. Childress (2018) provided scales that were said to assess relevant parent and child behavior and the extent to which it was normative, but did not provide any norms or any description of the way these scales were standardized. In a blog post (drcraigchildressblog.com), Childress has also described use of Pruter's Custody Resolution Method (CRM) a diagnostic approach which the present author has seen used in several reports in child custody cases. In his blog post, Childress states that CRM is based on a "data tagging methodology she uses for an archival data set (i.e. documented data; emails, texts, reports, court filings)" and which "is a standard methodology for compiling information from large sets of raw data" (drcraigchildressblog.com, Jan. 23, 2020). Childress, according to his blog and reports, then reviews the "data profile" and provides his opinion as a clinical psychologist. Childress (2015) also mentions his use of an ABAB design in which the, child's behavior is compared under treatment and no-treatment conditions and the comparison provides diagnostic information. A final point about identification of PA for this program is that children entering the program are generally court-ordered to attend and prohibited from contact with the preferred parent because the case is considered to involve PA.

A document thought to be written by Pruter (Conscous Co-Parenting Institute, n.d) describes events during the High Road program. This treatment closely resembles Family Bridges and uses one of the Family Bridges videos, "Welcome Back, Pluto", created by Warshak. Some children are brought to the treatment venue, a hotel or similar situation, by youth transport service workers. Children's phones, wallets, and IDs are taken away. The rejected parent is present and participates in treatment sessions. Children later go home with the rejected parent and have no contact with the preferred parent for at least 90 days.

According to Childress (2015), the High Road treatment is a "catalytic intervention" that "moves the child through a sequence of psychological states that deactivate the child's anxiety, restore the normal-range functioning of the child's empathy and attachment systems, and deactivate the child's inflamed anger" (p. 317)

Effectiveness

No systematic outcome study of High Road has ever been published. Childress (2015) notes that Pruter has reported a 100% success rate.

Potential harms

No research relevant to either benefits or harms of High Road has been published. In a case known to the present author, a child was diagnosed with and in treatment for PTSD following a High Road treatment.

Overcoming barriers family camp

Tenets

Overcoming Barriers is generally based on some assumptions shared with other intensive RTs, but also has as a foundation the view that children who reject a parent, and parents who are rejected, benefit from opportunities to work and play in a group, watch and listen to other families, and gradually move from observation into interaction. The focus of the program is on family conflict rather than PA alone.

Treatment methods

Children and parents are generally court-ordered to attend Overcoming Barriers after mental health professionals have recommended to the court that they need treatment for family conflicts and children's rejection of a parent. As is the case for other RTs, it is not known on what basis this decision is made. The Overcoming Barriers treatment involves a New England summer camp attended by children and both rejected and preferred parents. Recreational activities with parents, family meetings, and co-parent support groups are essential to the four days of Overcoming Barriers experiences.

Effectiveness

Saini (2019) conducted an on line survey of 40 parents who had attended Overcoming Barriers from six months to ten years previously. The focus of the survey appears to have been on the respondents' own feelings and on their interactions with the other parent. About half said that their conflicts with the other parent stayed about the same after the program, while about 25% said it got better. Other questions had similarly wide-ranging responses and did not allow clear conclusions. The relatively small number of participants, the length of time since some had taken part in the program, and the lack of any comparison group (even comparisons to the participants' opinions on entering the program) make any conclusions about the program's effectiveness quite uncertain.

Potential harms

Saini's (2019) survey of parents who had attended Overcoming Barriers was unusual and admirable in its consideration of possible unwanted outcomes. A substantial number of participants reported that their conflicts with the other parent and ability to problem-solve together got worse after the program. As was the case for effectiveness, possible harms done by the program cannot be ascertained in the absence of a comparison measure.

Transitioning families therapeutic reunification model

Tenets

Transitioning Families shares the assumptions of other intensive RTs and in addition assumes that experiential activities like swimming with dolphins and riding horses are important factors in improvement of parent-child relationships. There is stress on the importance of prohibiting contact with the preferred parent by court order and on building sanctions into those orders (Isicoff, 2015).

Transitioning Families is based on polyvagal theory (PVT) a formulation based on work by Stephen Porges (Porges, 2004; Porges & Furman, 2011). According to PVT, it is possible to link the state of the human autonomic nervous system (ANS) to social behavior, using information about the nervous system and about the evolution of the system from reptilian to mammalian forms. In the course of evolution, according to Porges, the addition of new structures and the modification of old ones led to new, adaptive social behaviors. "In this phylogenetically organized hierarchy [of three autonomic circuits], the newest circuit associated with social communication is used first [when threat is felt]. If that circuit fails to provide safety, the older survival-oriented circuits are recruited sequentially" (Porges & Furman, 2011, p. 109). The nervous system structure central to these events is the vagus (10th cranial nerve), which among other functions regulates heart rate. According to the PVT, it is possible to measure vagus nerve activity non-intrusively by a measure of heart activity called respiratory sinus arrhythmia (RSA).

PVT has received severe criticism from Grossman and Taylor (2007), who questioned the discussion of evolutionary effects on nervous system structures and commented unfavorably on the PVT description of ANS circuits. Grossman and Taylor suggested that changes in RSA are not reflections of emotional state, but instead have to do with regulation of energy exchange and synchronization of respiratory and cardiovascular processes.

The general concept of PVT can be challenged by reference to Grossman and Taylor (2007). Although Porges (2004) posits a Social Engagement System based on connections between the ventral vagus nerve and cranial nerves V (trochlear), VII (facial), IX (glossopharyngeal) and XI (spinal accessory), governing eye gaze, facial expression, and other social behaviors, he fails to note that two socially-important cranial nerves are omitted from this circuit. These are cranial nerve I (olfactory), responsible for the sense of smell that provides critical social cues for mammals, and cranial nerve VIII (auditory vestibular), essential to hearing and interpretation of vocal social cues of threat or safety. PVT claims may also be challenged on the absence of these nerves from the circuit that is posited to subtend social engagement.

Although there has been some discussion of the relevance of PVT to psychotherapy (e.g., Ryland et al., 2021), there has been little specific application of the theory to therapeutic work. However, Bailey et al. (2020) have provided an extensive discussion of the application of the PVT perspective in RT. As Bailey et al. note, although there are a number of treatment programs addressing children's contact resistance or refusal, none have received strong empirical support. Bailey et al. present their method's foundation in PVT as a supporting claim; arguments in favor of the use of this method can thus be challenged by reference to critiques of PVT such as the one by Grossman and Taylor, mentioned earlier.

Treatment methods

Children and parents are court-ordered to attend Transitioning Families. Bailey et al. (2020) presented an extensive description of Transitioning Families, and of its reliance on PVT principles. The work involves "neuroception", a term provided by Porges. According to Bailey et al., "not a cognitive process, neuroception is the way the ANS responds to cues of safety and danger felt inside the body, sensed in the environment, and signaled by other people" (p. 527). They propose that a primary goal of a PVT -based therapy is "to help clients recognize their states [and] find ways to move out of a numbed-out…or hyper-aroused … state and return to … the biological seat of safety and connectedness" (p. 530).

According to this approach, the therapist's job is to provide cues that help the client move from one state to another. A method for doing this, and helping the client become competent to manage states independently, is "mapping the ANS". The client is guided to use an image of a ladder, with the ventral vagal state of felt safety at the top, and other less desirable or comfortable states farther down. In the method suggested by Bailey et al., clients are asked to complete sentence the stems "I am…" and "The world is…" while in different states and later to use the language of their completions to refer to the way a state feels.

This aspect of Transitioning Families has a strong cognitive component, but other parts of the treatment focus on unconscious emotional and even directly physical treatments. For example, Bailey et al. approve of the use of equine-assisted therapies; these do not involve riding horses but working with them from the ground. According to Bailey et al.,

> horses can draw out a range of emotions and responses in families, which can then be used as therapeutic prompts for insight and directness… Because of this innate ability [of horses], horses are included as extensions of the therapeutic reunification team, and, as such, as agents of a therapeutic change (p. 535).

Bailey et al. suggest that other animals like dogs can take the place of horses in treatment, a suggestion contradictory to the findings of a feasibility study by Allen et al. (2021) on animal-assisted therapy.

In a practice they term psychoeducation, Bailey et al. teach parents and children "how to intentionally stimulate the ventral vagus to regulate the physiological response to the visceral perception of a sense of safety (neuroception). A few slow deep breaths from the belly, engaging the diaphragm (the stomach rises, not the chest), an extended exhalation, even just a sigh are ways to exercise the ventral vagus …" (p. 534).

Effectiveness

There is no published systematic outcome research on the effectiveness of Transitioning Families.

Potential harms

There are no published reports of harms caused by Transitioning Families.

Turning points for families

Tenets

In addition to assumptions shared with other intensive RTs, Turning Points stresses the idea that a child's rejection of a parent is "anti-instinctual" and therefore impossible in the absence of serious malevolent influence from the other parent. In supporting the possibility of parental alienation and the need for treatment, the founder of Turning Points, Linda Gottlieb says:

> ...our long dependency period depends upon a powerful instinct to need a parent—the child's survival is dependent on parents. *The need for a parent is therefore part of the instinct for survival* (italics *sic*). ...we crave connection with even an abusive parent in a process known as "undoing". It is only the intense brainwashing by the preferred or alienating parent that has the efficaciousness to overcome the child's powerful, self-protective, survival instinct to have and need a parent. (Gottlieb, 2021, p. 6)

Gottlieb's use of the term "instinct" reflects assumptions about the biological drivers of human behavior. Her reference to a long dependency period suggests the influence of evolutionary psychology (e.g., Cosmides & Tooby, 2013) with its stress on the inherited effects of human experiences in the environment of evolutionary adaptation (as John Bowlby termed it in his discussion of attachment). It is evident that the survival of young children depends on adult caregivers, but to say that there is an "instinct to need a parent" is hardly a meaningful statement, as a felt need stems from current experience rather than evolutionary history, and the term "instinct" has usually referred to heritable behaviors or behavior patterns. Gottlieb seems to state that an instinct, rather than a physiological state like hunger or fear, causes the felt need for a parent. She goes on to equate such a need with a posited "survival instinct".

Gottlieb's position on "instinct" as it shapes parent-child relations can be challenged on the basis of many published discussions of inheritance of behavior. Blumberg (2017), for example, commented on the use of terms like "survival instinct" and "maternal instinct". Such terms were many decades ago pointed out as simple attempts to retrofit motivations to observable behaviors, so if a creature survived, it was said to have a survival instinct; if it nurtured offspring, it was said to have a maternal instinct. Blumberg noted that

> these and other 'instincts' are not satisfactorily described as inborn, pre-programmed, hardwired, or genetically determined. Rather, research in this area teaches us that species-specific behaviors *develop* – and they do so in every individual under the guidance of species-typical experiences occurring within reliable ecological contexts. (p. 1)

Following this statement of Blumberg's, it is possible to challenge Gottlieb's claim that attachment to a parent is "instinctual", and rejection of a parent "anti-instinctual", by pointing out that behavior patterns result from a range of experiences acting in combination over time. The presence or absence of a given type of behavior does not indicate that a single damaging event has occurred (e.g. the experience of parental alienating behavior), but instead that behavior has been shaped by various combinations of experiences working on heritable characteristics.

It appears that Gottlieb's use of the "instinct" concept is not an effort to understand heredity and experience as they shape parent-child interactions, but involves the use of a commonly misunderstood term for the purpose of damning the posited "parental alienating behaviors", and identifying them as so viciously abusive that they can distort the emotions natural to the human species. Such identification should be challenged by consideration of current knowledge about behaviors characteristic of our species.

Treatment methods

Children attend Turning Points following a court order that also prohibits contact with the preferred parent for at least 90 days. They may be brought to the treatment venue by youth transport service workers. According to a description by Gottlieb (2021), children are to bring with them photographs or objects from their pre-divorce life with the rejected parent, to be used as evidence of the good relationship the parent and child once had. The four days of treatment are parallel with Family Bridges methods, including the use of the "Welcome Back, Pluto" video. Preferred parents are to attend therapy with Turning Points-approved practitioners and to write letters to the children explaining that the child's rejection of the other parent is entirely the fault of the preferred parent, who now regrets their actions. Gottlieb videotapes therapy sessions.

Effectiveness

Harman et al. (2022) collected data about TPFF, the intensive program run by the LCSW Linda Gottlieb. Like other PA interventions, TPFF requires that children be court-ordered into the program or that an agreement between the parents be approved by the court. Like other PA treatments, TPFF lasts about 4 days, involves prohibition of contact between child and preferred parent, for at least 90 days, and requires "aftercare" for both parents and child or children, performed by a a PA-approved therapist. TPFF also requires the preferred parent to write a letter to the child acknowledging his or her attempts at alienation. Gottlieb videotapes therapy sessions, and the videotaped material was made available to

Harman et al. Gottlieb, incidentally, claims almost 100% success in creating positive relationships between children and previously rejected parents; as this rate of success has been questioned, it was desirable from Gottlieb's viewpoint to have a positive report from Harman.

Harman and her colleagues were interested in evidence that TPFF was safe for children, as the present author and others have questioned whether this is so. On the grounds that none of the observed 32 children from 15 families ran away or carried out any self-harm during the program, and that Gottlieb states that none of the previously-treated children with whom she keeps in touch have done so, Harman concluded that TPFF was safe for children. She did not report on other possible aspects of harm, for example the PTSD diagnosed in a child following another PA intervention. Harman stated her belief that children who have reported distress and harm from PA interventions were simply still alienated, and would not have made such reports if their alienation had been repaired.

Harman also sought to know whether TPFF was an effective treatment for PA cases. To do so appropriately, of course, she would have needed to compare a group of TPFF-treated children with a matched control group who received no treatment or some other form of treatment. To compare behavior before and after treatment (as of course has also been done by Richard Warshak and other PA proponents) is to beg for confounding of variables so that it is impossible to know whether any changes were actually caused by the intervention. Reports following Family Bridges experience point to threats from therapists as reasons for behavior change (Barnett et al., 2022), but it is unknown whether such threats occur during TPFF.

Like some other PA proponents, Harman asked her staff to evaluate child behaviors on a Likert scale, rating behaviors from 1 to 5. Again like other PA proponents, Harman took these evaluative data and performed a statistical analysis which would only have been acceptable if the measurement method met certain criteria for parametric data, which were not met. The conclusion that TPFF is an effective treatment thus remains open to question.

There are many concerns about the basic data as well as about the data analysis. The videotapes evaluated by Harman's students were made by Gottlieb and certainly in her presence (it is not clear whether other people than parent and child were in the room at the time). This is far from an independent set of data, as Gottlieb's presence signaled to both parents and children what behaviors were desired, and indeed necessary to bring the program to an end. The correct method would have been to have the recording done by a person who was not aware of the purpose of TPFF and who observed parent and child without Gottlieb being present. Without wishing to stress that videorecordings can be cherry-picked, I would also note that the recordings should have stayed in the possession of the neutral recorder until handed over for analysis.

Harman et al. should be credited with attention to the possible harms associated with TPFF. However, they considered short-term harms like running away or self-harm as opposed to later anxiety, depression, or suicidality. In fact running away would not be easy, as TPFF, like other intensive RTs, takes away children's phones, money, and wallets. Self-harm would also be unusually difficult, as constant surveillance by a parent or the therapist makes it unlikely that razor blades or matches could be secreted by the child.

The research report by Harman, Saunders, and Afifi thus adds to the collection of weak studies of PA interventions, but in fact does not allow any clear conclusions about the safety or effectiveness of TPFF.

Conclusion

Many of the shared and specific tenets of RTs for PA are questionable. More importantly, the research evidence supporting the effectiveness of RTs has few strengths and many weaknesses. Without making the unreasonable demand that every psychological treatment meet criteria for EBT status, we must be aware that, at the minimum, outcome research is not acceptable unless the measures used have been established as valid and reliable, and unless in pre- and post-treatment designs the same measures are used before and after treatment. Leaving aside the many other issues like independent replication of RT outcome studies, mental health professionals and lawyers should note that this RT measurement problem means that "the best possible evidence" about RTs is not good enough to use for serious decisions affecting children and families.

When mental health principles and practices are offered as scientific evidence in court proceedings, they may be challenged as failing to meet standards for admissibility under *Daubert, Frye*, or other standards. Such challenges can be difficult either to mount or to respond to, as *Daubert* standards (for example) include the proviso that there be acceptance of the information by a relevant scientific community. The relevant scientific community for mental health issues consists primarily of researchers in the fields of psychiatry, psychology, and social work, who have for years struggled to define levels of evidence for complex mental health research topics (cf. Chambless & Hollon, 1998; "What is evidence-based treatment?", 2021). It may be as a result of these conceptual difficulties that challenges to the scientific admissibility of mental health outcome research are rare, and discussions about admissibility of specific information can be contentious (cf. Lorandos et al., 2020). The Association of Family and Conciliation Courts (AFCC) has posted relevant guidelines, with well-founded cautions about excessive generalization from social science research to individual cases (Association of Family and Conciliation Courts (AFCC),), 2018). Myers and Mercer (2022) have discussed approaches to challenging claims about parental alienation. In the opinion of the present author, claims made about RTs as of the date of this writing should also be challenged on grounds of scientific admissibility.

RTs are put forward as solutions to family problems involving children's resistance to or refusal of contact with a parent, and it would be premature to assume that they cannot function in that way. However, RT proponents have failed to make the case that they can identify and safely and effectively treat these problems, whether or not they actually involve parental alienation. The failure results from their lack of attention to detail, first and foremost, to measures of PA or other sorts of resistance, and subsequently, to high standards of research design and implementation.

Disclosure statement

The authors report no conflicts of interest. The authors alone are responsible for the content and writing of the paper.

ORCID

Jean Mercer http://orcid.org/0000-0003-3217-3953

References

Allen, B., Shenk, C. E., Dreschel, N. E., Wang, M., Bucher, A. M., Desir, M. P., Chen, M. J., & Grabowski, S. R. (2021). Integrating animal-assisted therapy into TF-CBT for abused youth with PTSD: A randomized controlled feasibility trial. *Child Maltreatment*, 107755952098879. https://doi.org/10.1177/1077559520988790

Association of Family and Conciliation Courts (AFCC). (2018). *Guidelines for the use of social science research*. https://www.afccnet.org.

Bailey, R., Dana, D., Bailey, E., & Davis, F. (2020). The application of the polyvagal theory to high conflict co-parenting cases. *Family Court Review*, *58*(2), 525–543. https://doi.org/10.1111/fcre.12485

Baker, A. (2005). The long-term effects of parental alienation on adult children: A qualitative research study. *American Journal of Family Therapy*, *33*, 289–302.

Barnett, A., Riley, A., & Katherine. (2022). Experiences of parental alienation interventions. In J. Mercer & M. Drew (Eds.), *Challenging parental alienation* (pp. 63–86). Routledge.

Blumberg, M. (2017). Development evolving: The origins and meanings of instinct. *Wiley Interdisciplinary Review of Cognitive Science*, *8*(1–2), e1371. https://doi.org/10.1002/wcs.1371

Bretherton, I. (1992). The origins of attachment theory: John Bowlby and Mary Ainsworth. *Developmental Psychology*, *28*(5), 759–775. https://doi.org/10.1037/0012-1649.28.5.759

Burbules, N., & Linn, M. (1988). Response to contradiction: Scientific reasoning durng adolescence. *Journal of Educational Psychology*, *80*(1), 67–75. https://doi.org/10.1037/0022-0663.80.1.67

Chambless, D., & Hollon, S. (1998). Defining empirically supported therapies. *Journal of Consulting and Clinical Psychology*, *66*(1), 7–18.

Childress, C. (2015). *An attachment-based model of parental alienation: Foundations*. Oaksong.

Childress, C. (2018). *An attachment-based model of parental alienation: Single case ABAB assessment & remedy*. Oaksong.

Conscious Co-Parenting Institute. (n.d.). *Overview of the high road to reunification program*. Unpublished document.

Cosmides, L., & Tooby, J. (2013). Evolutionary psychology: New perspectives on cognition and motivation. *Annual Review of Psychology*, *64*(1), 201–229. https://doi.org/10.1146/annurev.psych.121208.131628

Dimidjian, S., & Hollon, S. (2010). How would we know if psychotherapy were harmful? *The American Psychologist*, *65*(1), 21–33. https://doi.org/10.1037/a0017299

Garber, B., Prescott, D., & Mulcahy, C. (2021). *The family law professional's field guide to high-conflict litigation: Dynamics, not diagnoses*. ABA Publishing.

Gardner, R. (1985). Recent trends in divorce and custody litigation. *Academy Forum*, *29*(2), 3–7.

Gottlieb, L. (2021). *Turning points for families: A therapeutic vacation*. Unpublished paper. https://endparentalalienation.weebly.com.

Greenberg, L., Fidler, B., & Saini, M. (2019). *Evidence-informed interventions for court-involved families: Promoting healthy coping and development*. Oxford University Press.

Grossman, P., & Taylor, E. (2007). Toward understanding respiratory sinus arrhythmia: Relations to cardiac vagal tone, evolution, and biobehavioral functions. *Biological Psychology*, *74*(2), 263–285.

Harman, J., Saunders, L., & Afifi, T. (2022). Evaluation of the Turning Points for Families (TPFF) program for severely alienated children. *Journal of Family Therapy*, *44*(2), 279–298. https://doi.org/10.1111/1467-6427.123666

Isicoff, J. (2015). Reunification in parental alienation cases. Family Lawyer Magazine. https://familylawyermagazine.com/articles/reunification-in-parental-alienation-cases/

Lilienfeld, S. (2007). Psychological treatments that cause harm. *Perspectives on Psychological Science: A Journal of the Association for Psychological Science*, *2*(1), 53–70. https://doi.org/10.1111/j.1745-6916.2007.00029.x

Linden, M. (2013). How to define, find and classify side effects in psychotherapy: from unwanted events to adverse treatment reactions. *Clinical Psychology & Psychotherapy*, *20*(4), 286–296. https://doi.org/10.1002/cpp.1765

Lorandos, D., Lorandos, D., & Bernet, W. (2020). Admissibility of the construct—parental alienation. In C. C. Thomas (Eds.), *Parental alienation—Science and law* (pp. 365–385). IL.

Mercer, J. (2019). Are intensive parental alienation treatments effective and safe for children and adolescents? *Journal of Child Custody*, *16*(1), 67–113. https://doi.org/10.1080/15379418.2018.1557578

Mercer, J. (2021). Critiquing assumptions about parental alienation. Part 2. Causes of psychological harms. *Journal of Family Trauma, Child Custody, and Child Development*, *19*. https://doi.org/10.1080/26904586.2021.1957058

Mercer, J. (2022). Critiquing assumptions about parental alienation. Part I. The analogy with family violence. *Journal of Family Trauma, Child Custody, and Child Development*, *19*, 81–97.

Milchman, M. (2022). Distinguishing parental alienation from child abuse and adverse parenting. In J. Mercer & M. Drew (Eds.), *Challenging parental alienation* (pp. 107–137). Routledge.

Miller, S. (2022). How should alienated parents and their attorneys respond to false and misleading criticisms of alienation science? (Webinar). www.familyaccessfightingforchildrensrights.org.

Morris, S., Grice, J., & Cox, R. (2017). Scale imposition as quantitative alchemy: Studies on the transitivity of neuroticism ratings. *Basic and Applied Social Psychology, 39*(1), 1–18. https://doi.org/10.1080/01973533.2016.1256288

Myers, J., & Mercer, J. (2022). Parental alienation in family court: Attacking expert testimony. *Child and Family Law Journal, 10*, https://lawpublications.barry.edu/cflj/vol10/i1/3

Pietromonaco, P., & Barrett, L. (2000). The internal working models concept: What do we really know about the self in relation to others? *Review of General Psychology, 4*(2), 155–175. https://doi.org/10.1037/1089-2680.4.2.155

Porges, S. (2004). Neuroception: A subconscious system for detecting threats and safety. *Zero to Three, 24*(5), 19–24.

Porges, S., & Furman, S. (2011). The early development of the autonomic nervous system provides a neural platform for social behavior: A polyvagal perspective. *Infant and Child Development, 20*(1), 106–118.

Reay, K. (2015). Family Reflections: A promising therapeutic program designed to treat severely alienated children and their family system. *The American Journal of Family Therapy, 43*(2), 197–207. https://doi.org/10.1080/01926187.2015.1007769

Reichert, J., Richardson, J., & Thomas, R. (2015). Brainwashing": Diffusion of a questionable concept in legal systems. *International Journal for the Study of New Religions, 6*(1), 3–26. https://doi.org/10.1558/ijsnr.v6i1.22186

Ryland, S., Johnson, L., & Bernards, J. (2021). Honoring protective responses: reframing resistance in therapy using polyvagal theory. *Contemporary Family Therapy, 43*(2), 1–9.

Saini, M. (2019). Strengthening co-parent relationships to improve strained parent-child relationships: A follow-up study of parents' experiences of attending the Overcoming Barriers program. *Family Court Review, 57*(2), 217–230. https://doi.org/10.1111/fcre.12405

Trane, S., Champion, K., & Hupp, S. (2022). Comparison of parental alienation treatments and evidence-based treatments for children and adolescents. In J. Mercer & M. Drew (Eds.), *Challenging parental alienation* (pp. 138–158). Routledge.

Wadsworth, B. (2019). *Piaget's theory of cognitive and affective development* (5th ed.). Allyn & Bacon.

Warshak, R. (2010). Family Bridges: Using insights from social science to reconnect parents and alienated children. *Family Court Review, 48*(1), 48–80. https://doi.org/10.1111/j.1744-1617.2009.01288.x

Warshak, R. (2019). Reclaiming parent-child relationships: Outcomes of Family Bridges with alienated children. *Journal of Divorce & Remarriage, 60*(8), 645–667. https://doi.org/10.1080/10502556.2018.1529505

Warshak, R. (2020). Risks and realities of working with alienated children. *Family Court Review, 58*(2), 432–455. https://doi.org/10.1111/fcre.12481

"What is evidence-based treatment?" (2021). https://effectivechildtherapy.org.

How efficacious is Building Family Bridges? What the legal and mental health fields should know about Building Family Bridges and "parental alienation"

Diana S. Avalle, Brianna J. Smith, Katherine E. O. Wiedeman and Chris B. Garnica

ABSTRACT

Parental alienation (PA) has been defined as a situation when a child demonstrates a preference for one parent ("preferred parent") over the other ("targeted parent"). PA has become an influential topic in family courts and oftentimes programs like Building Family Bridges (BFB) are ordered because of the perceived impact of PA. There are concerns regarding methodological flaws in program research. Richard Warshak has become an influential proponent of BFB and has published articles suggesting it is a successful program. This publication addresses concerns of PA in courts, as well as BFB, that are based on junk science. This publication also provides judges with tools and information to utilize should cases involving allegations of PA arise in their courtrooms.

Parental alienation (PA) is a theory originally developed by psychiatrist Richard Gardner in 1985 (Gardner, 2008). This theory was first introduced as an opinion paper, not as a peer-reviewed research-based article. Dr. Gardner described PA as,

> A disorder that arises primarily in the context of child-custody disputes. Its primary manifestation is the child's campaign of denigration against the parent, a campaign that has no justification. The disorder results from the combination of indoctrinations by the alienating parent and the child's own contributions to the vilification of the alienated parent. (Gardner, 2008, p. 1)

It is said to exist when a child, without apparent reason, rejects a parent by refusing to see or talk to them (Haines et al., 2020). When PA is alleged, it is often said to have occurred due to one parent (the "preferred parent" [PT]) compromising the relationship between the child and the "targeted parent" (TP). This is said to occur as the result of one parent speaking negatively about the TP to the child, thus tarnishing the child's impression of the TP.

Parental alienation has been widely debated among the mental health, child advocacy, domestic violence, and legal communities and has become an influential topic in family court matters. A central criticism of PA being used in family courts is that PA proponents fail to acknowledge valid reasons for children favoring one parent, such as child abuse and/or domestic violence (DV), and instead solely focus on theories of the preferred parent influencing the child(ren). Circular reasoning is often used to argue that the preferred parent influences the child(ren) to make false allegations of abuse against the targeted parent, thus furthering the argument of severe PA. Research has demonstrated that when looking at false allegations of child sexual abuse, for example, a very small percentage (2–6%) are false allegations, and are typically made by the parent, rather than the child (Jones & McGraw, 1987). Not only can treating a child for misattributed PA invalidate a child's experience of abuse causing significant psychological harm, the misidentification of abuse may place children in danger, especially those that are then taken from a protective parent. As such, there is a distinct need to safeguard children against misattributed PA.

Despite many attempts by PA proponents, PA has been continually rejected as a disorder by the American Psychiatric Association (APA), among other major organizations, and thus it is not a formal medical or psychiatric diagnosis. Although the APA does not hold an opinion about the purported syndrome, they have stated, "An APA 1996 Presidential Task Force on Violence and the Family noted the lack of data to support so-called 'parental alienation syndrome' and raised concern about the term's use" (APA, 2008). Some PA proponents may use what are referred to as "V-Codes" (e.g., "Parent-Child Relationship problems") provided in the Diagnostic and Statistical Manual-5th edition (DSM-5) to categorize PA as a mental health or psychological concern. However, such V-Codes are not diagnoses; they are a means of providing additional clinical information for a given patient. The lack of reliable data to support the theory of PA in addition to the treatment programs claiming to treat PA have been a continued issue, which will be discussed here.

Reunification camps

It is believed by some that alienating behaviors by the preferred parent is a form of child abuse (Haines et al., 2020) and in some cases are addressed with what has been referred to as a "parentectomy" via "reunifications programs," also referred to as Parental Alienation Treatments (PATs) (Geffner & Sandoval, 2020; Mercer, 2019). PATs are programs that are often rooted in the theory of PA, and often have research on their effectiveness rates conducted by researchers who promote PA as well. BFB and the works by Warshak are no exception, which will be discussed further below. The ultimate goal of PATs is to reestablish the relationship between the child(ren) and the targeted parent. This is done typically by removing the child(ren) from the preferred parent completely and oftentimes granting full custody to the targeted parent.

While each PAT is unique in its program qualifications, treatment delivery, and requirements for being considered to have successfully completed the program, there are some universal truths in regard to how the PATs operate, and how they are researched. In many cases, the child(ren) is court-ordered to go to a retreat-like setting or a camp with the TP and is unable to have contact with the preferred parent. Meanwhile, the preferred parent is also required to participate in portions of the PAT geared specifically toward preferred parents thought to be influencing the child(ren) to think negatively about the TP.

Oftentimes PATs promote their services as "educational" and services are delivered, in part, by licensed clinicians; perhaps because not having a clinical diagnosis prohibits programs as advertising themselves as therapeutic in nature. The child(ren) is often presented with information on building critical thinking skills and problem-solving in order to undo the "brainwashing" from the preferred parent. After participating in the program, families are oftentimes encouraged, or mandated, to continued treatment with "aftercare programs." All the while, families are sometimes required to purchase various books and materials to supplement the in-person component. Because this is not promoted as a therapy-based intervention, it is not covered by insurance companies; therefore, it can become a lofty financial burden on a family as they are expected to pay out of pocket for these fee-for-service organizations. Additionally, although they are advertised as educational groups, rather than therapy-based groups, families are expected to pay fees for licensed mental health clinicians. While the programs are often promoted as lasting for up to two weeks, there have been cases in which they are required to participate for years due to resistance of children or preferred parent to meet exit goals, which will be discussed further below.

A central criticism of PATs is foundational in that it is not possible to accurately identify a child with PA against a child who does not "have" PA in order to do an accurate analysis of the effectiveness of interventions (Mercer, 2019). Because PA has been continually rejected by various medical and psychological governing bodies (e.g., American Psychiatric Association), there is no clinically-sound way to "diagnose" a case of PA, therefore, there is no way to accurately assess if PATs successfully "treat" PA. Secondly, many times PATs are court-ordered interventions, and because of the perceived resistance factor, often times children are transported to these facilities by workers who sometimes take the children away in handcuffs (Church, 2017). Many times PATs require the children be completely removed from the primary caretaker in order to best treat the perceived PA. Third, research has demonstrated that young adults who recalled any denigration of one parent by the other tended to feel negatively about both their parents, therefore rendering any notion of "brainwashing" moot (Mercer, 2019).

An issue and criticism of PAT research is that there are methodological concerns. These concerns include that there are no control groups with which to compare the children of the PATs to, there are no clearly defined outcome measures for program success, and nonrandom samples are utilized. Because randomized controlled or controlled clinical trials are not utilized, it is inaccurate to define the treatments as evidence-based. Additionally, the only measure often being evaluated are attitudes toward the TP (Mercer, 2019). There is no research on the specifics of the programs (e.g., reduction in PA "symptoms," increased critical thinking skills, etc.). These methodological concerns will be discussed further throughout.

Safety considerations

There are psychological safety issues to be taken into consideration. For example, as described above, PA may be used as a means of dismissing domestic violence children may have been subjected to or child abuse allegations. To have the custody arrangement reversed for participation in a PAT and force a child to live full time with the TP, who may be abusive, can be traumatic for that child. Research has demonstrated that children who experienced this reversal of custody to an abusive parent suffered from depression, PTSD, anxiety, self-harming behaviors and suicidality (Dallam & Silberg, 2016). Some children ran away from home which exposed them to other safety and trauma factors. The trauma of a high-conflict divorce may be exacerbated by these programs and not be in the best interest of the child(ren).

Building Family Bridges reunification program

A handful of PATs exist to treat a perceived case of PA, one such program being the Building Family Bridges (BFB) program. The BFB program was originally a result of the National Center for Missing and Exploited Children contacting a formerly licensed psychologist to develop a program to assist children who were fearful of their parents who had recovered them (Mercer, 2019). The irony of the origins of a PAT being for children who had been forcibly removed from their parents by a kidnapper, being the same means of "deprogramming" children supposedly suffering from PA is not lost on many PA criticizers. The BFB program is advertised to be a structured, educational four-day workshop that the TP participates in with their alienated child(ren). The advertised goal of BFB is to help children who hold negative, unrealistic attitudes toward a parent, and resist living with said parent, jump-start the recovery of a positive parent–child relationship by teaching better communication and conflict management skills. BFB claims to be appropriate for families when: a child has an unrealistic view of a parent; the child refuses contact with one parent or shows extreme reluctance to spend time with them; the family needs assistance transitioning to court orders that place the child(ren) in the sole custody of the TP; and when the child's negative attitudes and behaviors toward the TP are not reasonable or are not proportionate to that parent's behavior toward the child. It is noteworthy that parents cannot self-refer to the program. Referrals come through courts, child custody evaluators, therapists, attorneys or child representatives (e.g., guardian ad litems [GALs], or amicus attorneys).

Prior to enrollment in a workshop, families are required to schedule an initial 90-minute phone consultation for $500. Apart from this fee, additional costs associated with the workshop, as detailed above, are not advertised on the website. Additionally, BFB does not claim to provide therapy or counseling, asserting their workshop "provides an *educational* experience based on scientifically established concepts and procedures" [emphasis added] (Building Family Bridges, 2020). However, their website also notes that the workshops are led by licensed professionals who are regulated by their respective state boards.

Ethical issues concerning the BFB program

There are several legal and ethical considerations that have arisen regarding PATs. Notably, because they are often commercialized and trademarked, it is not possible to fairly evaluate them by independent researchers, as there is inaccessibility to trade secrets. Therefore, consumers (i.e., families and family courts) and researchers are left to formulate opinions and evaluate the programs based solely on the information provided by the organizations themselves. For example, one of the criticisms of BFB, along with other PATs, is that there is no information regarding training and qualifications for service providers of the program. The website does not advertise what types of credentials facilitators who are not mental health clinicians are required to obtain prior to becoming a "Family Bridges Workshop Provider." The only mention of this is that providers must undergo training in order to be authorized to provide BFB services; however, there is no mention of what exactly the training entails or how rigorous the vetting process is. Of additional concern is that those who have conducted the majority of the research on the efficacy of BFB are usually advocates of PA, which leaves one to question the integrity of such research, and if other independent researchers are granted access to data to do independent reviews.

The site goes on to outline the program's objectives which include: to help the child(ren) acclimate to a living situation with the "rejected" parent while ceasing contact with the "preferred" parent and (2) to enhance the relationship between the parent and child(ren). The intended goal of this program is to improve the quality of the parent-child relationship in just a span of four days. However, these objectives are rather subjective and do not have clearly defined outcomes that constitute success versus failure. For instance, the first objective intends to help the child(ren) adapt to being taken away from their "preferred parent," and many times primary custodial parent, in order to live with their "rejected parent." The BFB website reports that "Family Bridges has fulfilled one aim if, by the end of the workshop, the children are ready to return home with the rejected parent who has been awarded custody" (Building Family Bridges, 2020). This outcome is insignificant considering the child(ren) will often be forced to go home with the "rejected parent" regardless of their proclaimed readiness, as they have been court-ordered to do so.

Another critique specific to the BFB program is that the website-provided publications that support the efficacy of the workshop are primarily authored by the same individual. Thirteen out of the 17 publications provided are first authored by Warshak. This introduces the possibility of misleading the public regarding efficacy if the majority of the supportive publications are from one author. Additionally, many of the links to these publications for download take the reader to Warshak's website for the opportunity to purchase these publications along with books authored by Warshak. This suggests a symbiotic relationship between Warshak and the BFB program, as each benefit when the other does well. Basic research ethics suggest that a researcher should not directly benefit (monetarily or otherwise) from the groups, organizations, or subjects that they research. Additionally, a researcher who is intended to be a neutral party should not advertise programs he or she studies on their website.

Of particular concern to the mental health and child advocacy fields is that PATs appear, at times, to invalidate child(ren)'s experience and feelings. For example, the home page on the BFB website asserts, "Building Family Bridges helps children who resist living with a parent or hold unrealistic negative attitudes toward a parent" (Building Family Bridges,

2020). This statement provides support for BFB's invalidation with their assumption that the child(ren)'s beliefs are "unrealistic." The website does state, "Children whose rejection is reasonable, proportionate to and warranted by the history of the child's relationship with the rejected parent" would be ineligible for the BFB workshop; however, no operationalized definition is provided for what would be considered "reasonable" or "warranted" rejection (Building Family Bridges, 2020). Domestic violence and/or child abuse may be behind the child(ren)'s views; however, a determined history of such abuse may not be documented, as it is not uncommon for allegations of child abuse to be unsubstantiated, which does not necessarily equate to no abuse having occurred.

Anecdotal firsthand accounts of BFB experiences

There is growing anecdotal evidence of the coercive nature of some of the PATs from adults who were court-ordered to participate in various PATs during their childhood. Some individuals have made public statements via various media outlets (e.g., newspapers, podcasts, etc.). These reports highlight legal and ethical implications of a variety of PATs from beginning to aftercare programs. For example, some individuals have indicated that they were not allowed to eat until they said positive things about the TP (Martin, 2010). There are also statements suggesting that children are told if they do not say nice things about the TP, they will never be able to see the other parent or they will be incarcerated (Martin, 2010).

In one case recorded in a podcast, two teenage children were opposed to living with their mother, claiming she was emotionally and physically abusive (The Center for Investigative Reporting, 2019). After months of being ordered to "be nicer" to their mother, to bake with her, etc., the Judge grew frustrated. In a colloquy with the son, Alex, in chambers, the Judge said,

> You don't seem to get it, so I will tell you. I can send you, and you can cry. I can send you anywhere in this country and make you live anywhere, no father, no mother, no contact. You haven't done what I want you to do [be nice to his mother], and you are now gonna' have to rethink where you're going. (The Center for Investigative Reporting, 2019)

The Judge then sent Alex to juvenile detention to force him to change his attitude toward his mother (The Center for Investigative Reporting, 2019). When that did not work, the court ordered the family to participate in BFB, as recommended by the custody evaluator in the case. The children were instructed to turn over their phones and go with the police, who appeared at the door. They were not permitted to say good-bye or see their father and they were distraught after the Judge told them they would have to live with their mother and have no contact with their father for 90 days, despite the program being advertised as a four-day program.

The program took place in a hotel which the teenagers reported they were only allowed to leave for (supervised) meals. The daughter, Ana, reported her experience at BFB in this way: "[C]aptive is a good way to describe it. I felt watched all the time. I felt trapped." She reports that she and her brother were told "[they] couldn't leave the program until [they] said that [their] dad had brainwashed [them] [against the mother [they] said was emotionally abusive]." Finally, Ana reports, she got a "miraculous" two minutes alone with her brother, Alex, and told him:

> Alex, we need to fake it til we make it. This is legitimately the only way we are gonna get out of here. Whatever you think they'd want to hear, tell it to them. Just feed them anything that they want to hear. (The Center for Investigative Reporting, 2019)

In a second narrative reported in the podcast, a 14-year old girl begged the judge not to make her live with her mother, writing: "My mom screamed at me so much I started getting panic attacks. I wanted to kill myself just to make the pain go away. Please consider my needs and let me live with my father" (The Center for Investigative Reporting, 2019). According to the podcast, the child welfare agency had substantiated her claim of abuse. Nonetheless, the Judge involved in the case overrode the teen's description of her experiences and feelings and ordered her to a different reunification program, supposedly for five days. When her feelings toward her mother did not transform as a result of the staff's repeated insistence that her memories were untrue, they kept her there for 10 months, resulting in an invoice up an over $200,000. Ultimately, she was sent to boarding school by her mother (The Center for Investigative Reporting, 2019).

Warshak studies

Warshak has widely advocated for BFB's effectiveness in rebuilding and reforming parent-child relationships when PA is involved via self-conducted research. A variety of questionnaires and Likert-type ratings are used to track the progress of the parent-child relationships, the attitudes toward the program before and after participating, and the overall success of the workshop.

The empirical soundness of Warshak's research has been heavily criticized in the literature for similar reasons as outlined above. For example, as described above, selection for inclusion based on a child's resistance to contact with the rejected parent is inadequate given the lack of criteria to differentiate between children who are "alienated" and children whose resistance is based on their experience of abuse, destructive parenting, or exposure to domestic violence. Similarly, exit criteria based on statements that the program was helpful are meaningless without: assurance of free choice, any objective measures of the behavior changes in the parents or children associated with the improvement, sufficient information to objectively assess improvement in the parent-child relationship, and adequate safety and confidentiality of the responses at the conclusion of the intervention. Program evaluations based on global ratings of satisfaction do not provide enough specific information about how and why the program was helpful to be compelling, especially given the demand characteristics of the situation. Therefore, any reported results of program success appear overexaggerated and there lacks explanation of how or *if* these surveys were given in an anonymous and private fashion.

Some of Warshak's research studied children who were still in the custody of the TP, therefore, utilizing indeterminately anonymous surveys, further suggesting opportunity for coercive tactics on the part of the treatment team, evaluators, or parents. Without these explanations, it is possible that the entire context for the study provides strong cues to the children about pleasing the authorities who have control over them. These cues are consistent with the way Ana described her experience in the podcast discussed above. Warshak (2018) says the questionnaires were anonymous, but without more detail, any children who felt "captive" might not have trusted that the anonymity was real, as they were administered before the children had left the program. They were still under the watchful eye of the workshop leaders, as well as the parent the child did not want to be with. Children who may have felt coerced by those they perceived as captors might not trust whatever measures were taken to protect their anonymity. According to Warshak (2018), only 7% of the children said the program didn't help, but there is no information about who these children were and why they weren't satisfied. There is no way to know the percentage of the children who might have PA dynamics being misattributed to the family by courts or by misguided mental health professionals. Other research indicates that such errors do occur and that they are far from rare (Meier et al., 2019; Milchman, 2017; Silberg & Dallam, 2019). There is no way to know whether the reported 7% of dissatisfied children are the ones who alleged abuse or whether an unknown percentage of abused children were buried in the other 93% whose claim of satisfaction was a response to their feelings of coercion and the demand characteristics of the situation they were in.

Reviewing specific publications helps highlight the critiques provided above. In an initial study conducted in 2019, Warshak utilized a small sample to demonstrate BFB's goals, procedures, and effectiveness. In this sample of 23 previously "alienated" children from 12 different families, 22 were claimed to have restored a positive relationship with the parent they had rejected upon completion of the BFB workshop (Warshak, 2010). This was a specific sample of children who had supposedly been "alienated" for an average of more than two years from the rejected parent, 18 of whom maintained the positive relationships gained post-workshop for two to four years after attending according to Warshak (2010). It is noteworthy that four of the 22 children had "regressed" after the court allowed contact with the preferred parent again.

Another study utilized a sample size including four times as many families as in the aforementioned study and demonstrated comparable results (Warshak, 2018). Warshak claimed that of the 83 "severely alienated" children and adolescents that made up his sample, between 75–96% overcame the supposed alienation post-workshop. Additionally, Warshak reported that, "The percentage of children perceived as resisting compliance with the court-ordered contact with their alienated parent dropped from 85% before the workshop to 6% after the workshop according to the parents and 4% according to the workshop leaders" (Warshak, 2018, p. 16). This demonstrates that the success and progress of the workshop was measured by parent and professional perception of the child's behaviors and feelings, rather than the child's own reports, feelings, and statements. This brings to question the validity of the findings as "overcoming alienation" is not clearly defined, rather it is based on self-reporting of select participants. One is left to wonder why children's reports were not described here. Further results included parents rating the workshop, "even higher than did their children," with 75% of the parents rating it as, "excellent" and describing the relationship with their children as being, "much better." Important to note is that only 31% of the "alienated" children reported their relationship with the "rejected" parent as being, "much better" (Warshak, 2018).

In his claims, Warshak emphasized that the workshop itself did not harm children and justified the difference in reports from parent to children by stating, "according to the parents, [the workshop] was helpful even when a child did not appear to respond positively" (Warshak, 2018, p. 18). The results demonstrated that 15 of the children who participated in the workshop reported having 'somewhat negative' feelings about their experience, in which Warshak explained that, out of these 15 children, 12 had begun the workshop with already 'very negative' feelings thus the experience was, "not as bad as they had anticipated." It should be noted that often children walk into such programs with negative feelings about having to enter into such a program, hence why the program is being utilized in the first place. Warshak further justified these discrepancies by citing himself in a previous article stating that, "Children who remain alienated after the workshop are prone to complain about the experience, especially when aligned with the parent who opposed their participation in the workshop," (Warshak, 2018, p. 19). Rather than identifying this as a potential flaw, or area to be improved upon by the workshop itself, Warshak displaces the blame of program failures on the children.

Legal and ethical issues of Warshak and his studies

Warshak's claims that the BFB program is evidence-based raises questions about the legality and ethics of the program's efficacy. First, the BFB program is predicated on the presence of PA in the family system. However, because BFB has been criticized for lacking research regarding appropriate assessment criteria to accurately differentiate a child that is experiencing coercive parental favoritism from a child who is a victim of domestic violence, professionals and advocates alike are concerned with the severe negative impact of misattributed PA (Milchman et al., 2020). Specified rhetoric which impedes the empiricism of the opposing argument suggest that "false positives" exist within their assessments but fail to explore the enduring detriment their erroneous classifications have on such falsely identified children (e.g., Warshak, 2010, 2019). While both child custody and PA evaluators may often fail to accurately identify abuse where it is founded, the misidentification of abuse places children in the utmost danger, especially those who are then taken from a protective parent. As such, there is a distinct need to safeguard children against misattributed PA. Milchman and colleagues (2020) posit that a pressing safeguard against misattributed PA is to remove specific rhetorical devices from PA literature which misrepresent reasoning or evidence in order to make a compelling argument in their favor. Failure to accurately portray their "evidence" and to explore the possibility of genuine domestic abuse by establishing reliable and valid assessment criteria demonstrate gross negligence on the part of the program as well as ethical concerns regarding PA professionals' respect for persons, beneficence, and justice. The secretive, hidden dynamics of domestic violence are often overlooked, ignored, and used as a lack of evidence that such abuse has occurred.

Another major ethical concern, regards the safety and confidentiality for the respondents after the program concludes (Geffner, 2020). Geffner (2020) provides anecdotal examples of children who attended these programs as indications of coercion via firsthand accounts of reportedly falsified satisfaction, which Warshak uses as supportive data for BFB, although he may not necessarily be aware the accounts were falsified or reasons why the individuals may have felt compelled to do so. While these testimonials do not preclude the possibility of genuine satisfaction by some, they are substantial evidence of the inadequacy of the general satisfaction rating system, which as discussed above, may be a result of coercion or perceived potential for negative effects on the part of the children in the program. The authors are not aware of any published or substantive comments from Warshak in response to the criticisms of the evaluations.

While possible coercion, lack of anonymity, and fear of reproach lay an unethical foundation for the exit surveys, it is expressly concerning that BFB has incorporated these surveys into research without explicitly demonstrating that the research was approved by an Institutional Review Board (IRB) or aligned with the APA's Ethical Principles of Psychologists and Code of Conduct (American Psychological Association, 2017). As a psychologist, Warshak's (2019) research should adhere to his professional ethical standards, as outlined in the following:

> This Ethics Code applies only to psychologists' activities that are part of their scientific, educational, or professional roles as psychologists. Areas covered include but are not limited to the clinical, counseling, and school practice of psychology; research; teaching; supervision of trainees; public service; policy development; social intervention; development of assessment instruments; conducting assessments; educational counseling; organizational consulting; forensic activities; program design and evaluation; and administration. This Ethics Code applies to these activities across a variety of contexts, such as in person, postal, telephone, Internet, and other electronic transmissions. (APA, 2017, p. 2)

Relating to research, these codes state that psychologists must obtain institutional approval prior to conducting research (APA, 2017). Warshak's (2019) study cites that he is associated with the "Department of Psychiatry, Division of Psychology, University of Texas Southwestern Medical Center, Dallas, Texas, USA" (p. 1). Therefore, he should have sought approval from the institution's IRB prior to beginning the study. However, correspondence from the Division of Psychology Chief at the University of Texas Southwestern Medical Center (UTSW) in November of 2018 states although Warshak was previously a volunteer faculty, his appointment ended and no relationship between Warshak and the university existed at that time. Additionally, it is stated that UTSW "has not had involvement or oversight of any of Warshak's authored materials" (C.M. Cullum, personal communication, November 15, 2018). Therefore, it is unclear if Warshak has ever sought or obtained IRB approval before including human subjects in his research efforts, which could potentially put children at risk of psychological or physical danger, given the nature of his research.

The ethical code also notes that psychologists should avoid false or deceptive statements, including avoiding "false, deceptive, or fraudulent statements concerning ... their institutional or association affiliations," (APA, 2017, p. 8). If Warshak was not affiliated with UTSW, nor obtained an IRB approval, it would raise ethical concerns about the research and for any publications. The article made no mention of informed consent, protection of human participants, or precautions for reducing or eliminating researcher bias and expectancy effects. Warshak's claims that the BFB program is evidence-based may exhibit unethical professional practices until such a time that he can produce evidence to the contrary.

Conclusion

Parental alienation is a concept that will likely be disputed for years to come, as this terminology is entrenched in the court system and can be used as a divisive explanation in divorce and child custody cases. It is important to understand the full scope of issues associated with attaching the term "parental alienation" to any person, family, treatment program, clinician, or researcher. Parental alienation continues to be rejected as a disorder, therefore, claims of evaluating those who "have it" and providing treatment to child(ren) and families are essentially speculative. As such, jurisdictions that are to adhere to the Daubert standard should consider whether PA-based testimony (including PATs) are inadmissible due to its lack of reliable and valid ways of assessing and determining its presence as this standard requires that any expert testimony (e.g., testimony to substantiate the effectiveness of camps such as BFB in family court cases) should be based, in part, on "reliable principles and methods" (Mueller et al., 2018).

Additionally, safety issues can arise, as many child(ren) are forced to attend PATs while neglecting to acknowledge domestic violence and/or child abuse situations the child(ren) may have been exposed to. Overgeneralization, and an eager inclination to pathologize PA, can result in a disregard to identify actual abuse taking place.

From a research efficacy standpoint, research on many treatment programs, such as BFB, cannot be performed by those who are so closely connected and demonstrate a symbiotic relationship, such as Warshak. This creates an opportunity for biased results. Without allowing those outside of the organization to conduct research, an invitation exists to create duplicitous literature around PA. This also leads to the implementation of treatment programs with steep price tags, under the guise of a desired result for the families.

It can be difficult for family courts to sift through the volumes of literature out there both for and opposed to PA or PATs. However, it is possible to do a thorough examination of any family court involved case in which PA and/or abuse are being alleged. In cases in which PA is alleged, it is of utmost importance to understand the dynamics of power and control that are often present in domestic violence. As such, any cases in which PA is being alleged, a comprehensive evaluation to screen for child abuse and/or domestic violence is advised. This can and should be done by a neutral, third-party evaluator who is well-versed in domestic violence. Additionally, family courts can benefit from examining the legal and ethical issues outlined in this article to assess the validity of mental health professionals who may be touting PA-based theories and concepts. Oftentimes children's voices are overshadowed by all the adults involved in such cases, that their perspectives and experiences are not seen or heard and in situations in which they are heard, their statements are used against them as further "evidence" of PA, rather than looking at such statements objectively.

Acknowledgments

We would like to acknowledge and thank Robert Geffner for his contributions to this publication.

Disclosure statement

None of the authors have any disclosures of conflict to report.

Ethical standards and informed consent

No human subjects were involved in the development of this article.

References

American Psychological Association. (2017). *Ethical principles of psychologists and code of conduct*. Author.

American Psychological Association. (2008, January 1). Statement on parental alienation syndrome [Press release]. https://www.apa.org/news/press/releases/2008/01/pas-syndrome

Building Family Bridges. (2020, August 31). Frequently asked questions. https://buildingfamilybridges.com/faqs/

Church, L. R. (2017, September 4). Taken from mom, teen flees dad and waits for 18th birthday. *Livingston Daily*. https://www.livingstondaily.com/story/news/local/community/livingston-county/2017/09/04/parent-alienation-bill/589157001/

Dallam, S., & Silberg, J. L. (2016). Recommended treatments for "parental alienation syndrome" (PAS) may cause children foreseeable and lasting psychological harm. *Journal of Child Custody*, *13*(2–3), 134–143. https://doi.org/10.1080/15379418.2016.1219974

Gardner, R. A. (2008). Parental divorce and the needs of children. *Family Court Review*, *13*(2), 1–5. https://doi.org/10.1111/j.174-1617.1975.tb01335.x

Geffner, R. (2020). Critique of Warshak's research on Family Bridges program. Unpublished manuscript.

Geffner, R., & Sandoval, A. (2020). Parental Alienation Syndrome/Parental Alienation Disorder (PAS/PAD): A critique of a 'disorder' frequently used to discount allegations of interpersonal violence and abuse in child custody cases. *APSCA Advisor*, *32*(1), 28–37.

Haines, J., Matthewson, M., & Turnbull, M. (2020). *Understanding and managing parental alienation: A guide to assessment and intervention*. Routledge, Taylor & Francis Group.

Jones, D. P., & McGraw, J. M. (1987). Reliable and fictitious accounts of sexual abuse to children. *Journal of Interpersonal Violence*, *2*(1), 27–45. https://doi.org/10.1177/088626087002001002

Martin, S. T. (2010, May 23). Parental alienation: Sickness or psych job? *Tampa Bay Times*. https://www.tampabay.com/archive/2010/05/23/parental-alienation-sickness-or-psych-job/

Meier, J. S., Dickson, S., O'Sullivan, C., Rosen, L., & Hayes, J. (2019). Child custody outcomes in cases involving parental alienation and abuse allegations. *GWU Law School Public Law Research Paper* (2019-56). https://ssrn.com/abstract=3448062

Mercer, J. (2019). Are intensive parental alienation treatments effective and safe for children and adolescents? *Journal of Child Custody*, *16*(1), 67–113. https://doi.org/10.1080/15379418.2018.1557578

Milchman, M. S. (2017). Misogyny in New York custody decisions with parental alienation and child sexual abuse allegations. *Journal of Child Custody*, *14*(4), 234–259. https://doi.org/10.1080/15379418.2017.1416723

Milchman, M. S., Geffner, R., & Meier, J. S. (2020). Ideology and rhetoric replace science and reason in some parental alienation literature and advocacy: A critique. *Family Court Review*, *58*(2), 340–361. https://doi.org/10.1111/fcre.12476

Mueller, C., Kirkpatrick, L., & Richter, L. (2018). *Evidence §7.7§7.7 Reliability Standard (Daubert, Frye)* (GWU Law School Public Law Research Paper No. 2018-71; GWU Legal Studies Research Paper No. 2018-71. *SSRN*. https://ssrn.com/abstract=3277067

Silberg, J., & Dallam, S. (2019). Abusers gaining custody in family courts: A case series of over turned decisions. *Journal of Child Custody*, *16*(2), 140–169. https://doi.org/10.1080/15379418.2019.1613204

The Center for Investigative Reporting. (2019, March 9). Bitter custody. *Reveal* [Podcast]. https://revealnews.org/podcast/bitter-custody/

Warshak, R. A. (2010). Family Bridges: Using insights from social science to reconnect parents and alienated children. *Family Court Review*, *48*(1), 48–80. https://doi.org/10.1111/j.1744-1617.2009.01288.x

Warshak, R. A. (2018). Dr. Richard Warshak. https://www.warshak.com

Warshak, R. A. (2019). Reclaiming parent-child relationships: Outcomes of Family Bridges with alienated children. *Journal of Divorce & Remarriage*, *60*(8), 645–667. https://doi.org/10.1080/10502556.2018.1529505

The "solution" to parental alienation: A critique of the turning points and overcoming barriers reunification programs

Elena Andreopoulos and Alison Wexler

ABSTRACT
Parental alienation is a phenomenon in psychology that has garnered tremendous controversy over the past sixty years (Joshi, 2021). Especially within the realm of high-conflict divorce cases, parental alienation is considered by some mental health professionals as a great concern that can be resolved through reunification therapy or related educational programs. These educational programs, which aim to bring families together and attempt to rectify the concern of parental alienation, are seen in Linda Gottlieb's *Turning Points* (New York, New York; Austin, Texas) as well as Deutsch, Ward, Sullivan, and Friend's *Overcoming Barriers* (Palo Alto, California; Natick, Massachusetts; New York, New York). In this paper, we highlight research findings of the programs, methods used, limitations, as well as critiques of the programs. Ultimately, there is a lack of reliable research behind each of these programs and a potential concern for traumatizing individuals who engage in such programs.

The notion that divorce establishes circumstances where a distressed parent might attempt to turn a child against the other parent is not novel. For almost 200 years, people have heard terms such as "poisoning the child's mind" and "alienating the child's affection" used in legal cases (Lorandos et al., 2013). Parental Alienation (PA) refers to the child's strong alliance with one parent and rejection of a relationship with the other parent without legitimate justification (Bernet, 2010). This has led to the term in psychological research and published literature known as Parental Alienation Syndrome (PAS). Although a more complex concept, Parental Alienation Syndrome refers to a child with parental alienation who manifests some or all of eight characteristic behaviors. These eight behaviors include: the child's campaign of denigration against the alienated parent; frivolous rationalizations for the child's criticism of the alienated parent; lack of ambivalence; the independent-thinker phenomenon; reflexive support of the preferred parent against the alienated parent; an absence of guilt over exploitation and mistreatment of the alienated parent; borrowed scenarios; and spread of the child's animosity toward the alienated parent's extended family (Gardner, 1992a). PA refers to the alienating behaviors of a parent. PAS are symptoms manifested by the child (Darnall, 2011).

Parental alienation researchers and advocates believe such dynamics and symptoms can be resolved through psycho-educational interventions for alienated children, reunification therapy for alienated children and rejected parents, or even co-parenting classes to reduce parental conflict (Lorandos et al., 2013). The most commonly applied approach would be reunification therapy. Reunification therapy is a recently developed therapeutic modality for treating high-conflict, litigious families (Darnall, 2011). The purpose of the reunification therapy when PA is purported to be present is to encourage a change in the child's attitudes (Lorandos et al., 2013). The focus of the therapy is reportedly encompassed into three components: tempering the hostilities of the alienating parent; assuring an emotional and safe environment for the children with both parents and significant others; and repairing the damaged relationships with the children (Darnall, 2011). However, this is one way reunification therapy can be applied, as it can also be practiced outside of supposed PA cases.

There are several programs across the United States of America that attempt to address issues of Parental Alienation through reunification therapy. Some of the most notable programs in this discipline are Deutsch, Ward, Sullivan, and Friend's *Overcoming Barriers* (OCB; located in Palo Alto, California; Natick, Massachusetts; New York, New York) and Linda Gottlieb's *Turning Points* (TPFF; located in New York, New York and with a branch in Austin, Texas run by Loretta Maase). Although these programs have gained a following through various cases of high conflict divorces, there are several concerns and a persistent lack of reliable research that substantiate the methods used in the practices of the programs. In this paper, we will thoroughly detail and analyze the literature surrounding each program, their methods, summary of findings, limitations, critiques, and suggested points of future thought.

Linda Gottlieb's Turning Points

Located in New York, Linda Gottlieb's website Turning Points program states it is a "short-term, effective treatment program to restore healthy family functioning between parent and child and to promote a civil and respectful co-parenting relationship" (Gottlieb, 2021b). Turning Points for Families (TPFF) is a four-day, transitional program to "jump-start" the healing of a severed or severely damaged relationship between a child and parent. According to Gottlieb and the Turning Points Program's website, parental alienation refers to:

> An observable family dynamic in which a child denigrates and rejects a parent (known as the alienated parent) in the absence of a reasonable or valid reason—child abuse/neglect or a pattern of markedly deficit parenting—and justifies the rejection with weak, trivial, frivolous, or absurd reasons (Gottlieb, 2021a, p. 1).

Gottlieb states the influencing parent, also known as the alienating parent, "manipulates the child through a brainwashing process to sever or severely undermine the relationship between the alienated parent and child" (Gottlieb, 2021a, p. 1).

Affiliated literature

Linda Gottlieb believes such dynamics can be resolved through reunification therapy and research demonstrates the effectiveness of this approach. According to Gottlieb, research shows relapse is certain if the child were to have contact with the "unreformed alienating parent" (Gottlieb, 2021a, p. 6). Gottlieb has written and published two works on parental alienation, a book as well as a book chapter (Gottlieb, 2012, 2013). Gottlieb has also written several pieces on topics and scenarios related to parental alienation. These works are not published in academic journals nor do not appear to have undergone the official peer review process. The two prominent works featured on the Turning Points website are entitled *Children are Harmed when Professionals Reject Science* (Gottlieb, 2020a) and *Reasons for the Apology Letter from The Alienating Parent* (Gottlieb, 2020b). In the first work, Gottlieb discusses being "stunned" by the "exceedingly high number" of professionals who come to believe the false abuse allegations, as reported by the child, are true (Gottlieb, 2020a, p. 2). Research has consistently shown children typically tell the truth and false allegations only represent a small percentage of the population (Faller, 1984; Lyon & Dorado, 2008; O'Donohue et al., 2018; Ruck, 1996; Rush, 2014). Gottlieb states she is "unaware of any peer-reviewed studies on the prevalence of the phenomenon of false child abuse allegations in alienation cases" and proceeds to provide statistics based on her experiences in her practice (Gottlieb, 2020a, p. 2). According to Gottlieb (2020a), from having treated 700 children who were victims of alienation to some degree, 80% (550) of the moderate to severe cases of PA had made at least one knowingly false child abuse allegation. Gottlieb does not operationally define what she classifies as moderate or severe cases of PA. It is important to ponder how accurate these statistics are reported to be without a research study conducted at the time of writing. The validity and generalizability of these results is a source of concern. Gottlieb (2020a) states parental alienation is especially of great concern when a child sex-abuse allegation is made as it could have serious consequences in the family dynamic. Gottlieb (2020a) refers to the substantial peer-reviewed research on the suggestibility of children, particularly mentioning research by Dr. Julia Shaw and Dr. Elizabeth Loftus. By mentioning these findings, Gottlieb infers to the notion that children can be susceptible to making false allegations when "coached" by the alienating parent. Although this research was popularized in the 1980s and 1990s, current research trumps prior findings of suggestibility research and demarks such prior research as outdated by not having considered the length of the suggestibility. Research has found individuals can forget the false details after a prolonged period and it is uncommon for an allegation to derive from coaching (Brainerd & Poole, 1997; Chan et al., 2022; Faller, 2007; Starns & Hicks, 2005). If one considers a child custody case, high conflict divorce, or a family sex-abuse allegation, the child would be asked to repeat their version of events repeatedly over several months to various professionals. As a result, false allegations would be very difficult to uphold throughout these different evaluations.

In the second aforementioned piece, Gottlieb argues alienated children know they have abused/maltreated/rejected a parent and they suffer guilt for their entire lives as a result unless they are fully exonerated of these behaviors (Gottlieb, 2020b). She states children might not immediately recognize and acknowledge their abusive parent, but they will be adversely affected when they eventually come to recognize it (Gottlieb, 2020b). Gottlieb cites the research of Amy Baker (Baker & Fine, 2007) regarding the concept of guilt in alienated children. Gottlieb explains that for the exoneration cycle of the child's guilt to be completed, "the alienating parent must accept full responsibility for the child's rejection and maltreatment of the alienated parent" (Gottlieb, 2020b, p. 1). To teach children to take responsibility for their mistakes is to model taking responsibility for their behaviors. Gottlieb proposes this be done through an apology letter for causing the alienation and emphasizing the alienated parent had not abused them nor placed the child at risk as well as apologizing for "having created… such distortions, untruths, and utterly fabricated allegations of child abuse" (Gottlieb, 2020b, p. 3). This apology is meant to reduce the child's risk potential for dysfunction across behavioral, cognitive, emotional, and interpersonal domains. Within the text, it is not considered how one can distinguish between false or truthful accusations. Additionally, it may be important to consider how the child would feel about the "alienating parent." This is vital to consider as it could influence the entirety of the family dynamic and not solely the relationship between the child and the "alienated" parent.

Method

Participants

There is not a substantial amount of information regarding the parents or families that have participated in the Turning Points for Families program. Gottlieb states families eligible for TPFF are referred by the court and must have an order that includes program engagement, interventions, and specific custody arrangements (Gottlieb, 2021a, p. 14–15).

There are nine testimonials on the Turning Points program website, mainly from fathers who have been accused of abuse; however, there is no information regarding the families who have engaged in the program. As of the TPFF program assessment conducted by Harman and colleagues, the main information is participants mainly come from the United States of America and likely attain good financial standing (Harman et al., 2021).

Procedures

The program operates on the idea that the court has determined "(1) the child is safe in the care of the [alienated] parent, and (2) the [alienating] parent has, at a minimum, interfered with and/or not adequately supported the relationship between the other parent and their child" (Gottlieb, 2021a, p. 11). However, TPFF is considered "not suitable for and does not accept referrals for cases of bona fide protective causes for the rejection" (Gottlieb, 2021a, p. 11).

The program consists of a three to four-hour therapy session which is provided daily each of the four days. The rest of the day consists of the "rejected" parent and child engaging in "continual new corrective experiences" with each other (p. 14). They do this by exploring the local attractions and experiencing common interest activities in New York City. Gottlieb suggests they can visit the local library, where the "rejected" parent can tutor the child if needed. They can also engage in other activities such as going to museums, amusement parks, toy stores, gardens, swimming, boating, bowling, ice-skating, hiking, rock climbing, and trampolines.

Throughout the four days, Gottlieb provides a specific procedure for the family to undergo. During the first day, Gottlieb explains she asks the "alienated" parent to bring any pictures or videos of their children and she "walks them down memory lane" (Long Island Backstory, 2018).

Gottlieb takes them to lunch and then the afternoon activities begin. Gottlieb takes pictures of the parent and child engaging in the activities and sends them to the "alienating" parent. Gottlieb claims that she takes these pictures and videos for purposes of the court as well as to demonstrate body language and affect which cannot be emphasized enough in a report. The intended purpose of this engagement is so that the "rejected" parent's authority with the child is reestablished through the supervision, nurturing, and support being provided by her or him throughout the four days. Linda Gottlieb herself accompanies the family on these activities. According to her, Gottlieb coaches and intervenes, when necessary, as well as monitors the developments. On the second day, Gottlieb has the child and the "alienated" parent watch *Welcome Back, Pluto* (Long Island Backstory, 2018). This video is meant to show the typical story of what an "alienated" parent has to go through. On day three, Gottlieb educates the child and the "alienated" parent on the "ease of implanting memories and distorting memories" (Long Island Backstory, 2018). On the last day, Gottlieb discusses a summary of what occurred, and the child goes home with the "formerly alienated" parent. Gottlieb states that the alienating parent does not participate. The alienating parent is asked to write a letter to the child stating: "I support the reunification and this is why, these are the qualities your other parent has to offer you, and this is why you need your other parent meaningfully in your life". Gottlieb explains "unfortunately, most alienators [are] not able to write that letter" and "the letter is a *test* to determine the resolve of the alienating parent, but it is not needed for reunification" (Long Island Backstory, 2018). The notion that most "alienators" are unable to compose such a letter suggests treatment is typically not fully accomplished, and this part of the program is quite unsuccessful.

Ultimately, the family sees a family therapist which Gottlieb collaborates with and there must be a 90-day no contact period with the alienating parent (Long Island Backstory, 2018).

The success of this program relies on the 90-day no contact period with the alienating parent to be adhered to. Gottlieb explains that after the program, the family's engagement with an "experienced family therapist assures maintenance and enhancement of the reunification" (Gottlieb, 2021a, p. 17). Gottlieb does not recommend individual therapy follow-up therapy for the child, stating it is generally forbidden and individual therapy for the child "will only serve as a forum for the programmed child to revert to venting the programmed script, just as a cult member will only repeat the words of the cult leader" (Gottlieb, 2021a, p. 18). The concern arises as to whether the child is provided space to express and discuss their feelings or thoughts.

Several concerns arise as a result of the program's procedures. First, there is no method proposed by Gottlieb to detect legitimate abuse from the "alienated" parent. Although the court would have determined no abuse presence, Gottlieb would ideally have her own procedure of evaluating these circumstances. Gottlieb has stated that even if there is no alienation, "there is no downside to the program as it is time with the other parent" (Long Island Backstory, 2018). Without a procedure in place, there is an increased risk of the child being at the hands of the "alienated" parent. It is also not specified if Gottlieb and her team administer any scientific or psychological measures with the family during their engagement. Knowing such information would aid in determining the scientific validity or reliability of the program's outcomes.

Second, the accommodations are not paid for by the program. Considering this program is located in New York City, it is important to note that the necessary accommodations to partake in the program, and the program itself, would be costly. Unfortunately, there is no indication on the website as to the cost of the program and it is unclear if the suggested outdoor activities are included in the overall cost. Based on some of the court orders Gottlieb made available online, it could be that the cost is approximately $6,000 per parent. This lack of transparency can be seen as concerning, as it is unclear how much families are being charged and whether or not this is considered a reasonable price for the work that is being completed in the program.

Results

According to Gottlieb, Turning Points has proven to be a highly successful reunification program. On the program's website, Gottlieb states they have "maintained statistics and data for several criteria regarding the program's outcomes; the psychological, cognitive, and behavioral improvements of the child; and the removal from the alienating parent and placement with the alienated parent do not traumatize the child" (Gottlieb, 2021a, p. 15). The concern was we did not see any of these findings available on the website. According to Gottlieb, outcome data and effectiveness of the Turning Points intervention were "in process of being assessed and evaluated by the Colorado State University both for its success of reunification and the positive effect on the alienated child" (Gottlieb, 2021a, p. 15). It was mentioned "the analysis [was] expected to be completed in early to mid-2020 and expected to be published in a peer-reviewed journal" (Gottlieb, 2021a, p. 15).

As the time frame had passed, the authors thought it valuable to contact Linda Gottlieb and her team regarding the publication of this evaluation.

The program administrator noted that they "expect the review to be really good and can't wait till it is done". Dr. Harman, who also replied, stated that the evaluation was set to be completed soon, as COVID slowed things down quite a bit. However, at the time, the results of the analyses and preparation for publication were underway. The paper was to be submitted for review sometime toward the middle or end of January 2021 and take weeks to months to go undergo the peer review process. The authors also contacted Loretta Maase from the Austin, Texas branch of the Turning Points program to understand what kind of research or statistics of program effectiveness were available. She explained that "the only official research to date will be a study by Dr. Jennifer Harman at the University of Colorado." She said she would be happy to let the authors know when the research is published and that it would show that the "Turning Points program has a success rate of approximately 98% when treatment protocols are followed (90-day no contact)."

Within the context of research, it is not typical to know the results of the study before the analysis is conducted. During the initial stages of correspondence, prior to the study being published, there was a concern regarding the possible biased nature of this study as well as the validity of its conclusions. The individual conducting the study, Dr. Jennifer Harman, is also a leading researcher in the field of Parental Alienation. For a scientifically unbiased review, the main reviewer should have been neutral to the position in question. If not, then at least it would have been imperative to have multiple researchers weigh in on the review to have various perspectives vocalized in the evaluation. This could have happened via the process of peer-review and therefore the authors could not assume this was not going to occur.

The study was officially published on September 7, 2021, the delay of publication likely due to the global pandemic (Harman et al., 2021). Dr. Jennifer Harman's study, *Evaluation of the Turning Points for Families (TPFF) program for severely alienated children*, was co-written with graduate student Luke Saunders (Colorado State University) and professor of communications, Dr. Tamara Afifi (University of California Santa-Barbara). Findings demonstrated 96.4% of fifty-five children reconnected with the alienated parent as a result of the TPFF program (Harman et al., 2021). Results revealed TPFF was found to be a safe program for children and that "participants in the TPFF program either had positive changes, or their ratings on the scales remained stable (i.e. no significant negative changes) over time" (Harman et al., 2021, p. 13).

The study at first glance appears to be a thorough examination of data of families who participated in the TPFF in the past (Harman et al., 2021). First, Harman and her colleagues were able to provide a comprehensive literature review of the concept of parental alienation, along with research of programs similar to TPFF. The authors also provide a detailed description of the TPFF program as well as what each day entails (Harman et al., 2021). Second, there was an attempt to minimize some bias in the study, by including professionals who were not familiar with TPFF. Both the colleagues that she co-wrote the article with, as well as those who were assigned to code the TPFF data, were reportedly not familiar with the program (Harman et al., 2021). Nevertheless, there still is a significant bias with the first author of the study, Dr. Jennifer Harman, who is a leading researcher and advocate in the field of parental alienation. Third, the data were de-identified and made public such that other researchers could access it. This access to the data is important as others can have a better understanding of how these data look and can be analyzed (Harman et al., 2021). Lastly, it is beneficial that Harman and her colleagues address the issues regarding the cost of the program. Harman notes that the program may be "financially unobtainable for many families in need of intervention for severe parental alienation" and the "findings may not generalize to families that lack the means to participate" (Harman et al., 2021, p. 17). Although the average cost of the program is never mentioned in the article, the awareness that the program's cost makes it inaccessible to some is a very important limitation to acknowledge.

The study itself has a multitude of issues regarding the overall research design and subsequent analysis. The critique of this first and only research conducted about TPFF is best presented by Dr. Jean Mercer, professor emerita at Stockton University. As discussed in Dr. Mercer's blog *Child Myths*, Harman and colleagues demonstrate issues with the study design regarding levels of evidence, measurement, severity as well as their implications for research design, and harm (Mercer, 2021b).

The primary concern of the study lies with the validity behind the ultimate conclusion that TPFF is an effective treatment. When conducting a study regarding the effectiveness of a treatment, a proper conclusion can only be made when "the outcome research has involved randomized controlled trials or careful clinical controlled trials" (Mercer, 2021b). The group of individuals who underwent the treatment would need to be compared to similar individuals who received a different treatment or no treatment at all. In doing so, one can then make a more evident conclusion regarding the differences and impact the treatment had on people as opposed to people who received a different treatment or no treatment. By lacking the presence of these control groups, it is difficult and misguided to conclude that the TPFF program is more effective than engaging in another treatment or no treatment over time. As a proponent of parental alienation, Dr. Harman could have a vested interest in demonstrating that a reunification program is effective, as it would validate the concept of parental alienation and Gottlieb's program would have a peer-reviewed study to refer to for the courts as well as the families involved. What would be the incentive or benefit of hypothesizing and finding this program could be unsuccessful?

As Dr. Mercer points out, the secondary concern lies in the measurements utilized in the study (Mercer, 2021b). The quantitative analyses conducted are not considered with the appropriate statistical procedures. The ratings of participants in the TPFF programs are not considered properly due to the statistical procedures used, as Likert scale ratings cannot be applied in arithmetical operations which are needed for parametric statistics. Harman expressed that they "did not anticipate large changes in relationship quality in a short, 4-day intervention" (Harman et al., 2021, p. 12). As Mercer notes, if one does not anticipate a great change in 4 days, one should also explore what is the purpose a 4-day intervention (Mercer, 2021b). It could be argued that the therapeutic work continues after the 4-days; nevertheless, it is difficult to measure the proper effectiveness of the program even without control groups.

Mercer also delves into the notion of "severity" in these cases of parental alienation (Mercer, 2021b). Harman states that in the sample many of the children and alienated parents made significant progress toward reunification before participation in the TPFF program (Harman et al., 2021, p. 12). If this is the case, one should consider how "severe" these cases were and how exactly this is operationalized by Gottlieb's program, in addition to the findings from the court. Given this prior "significant progress" between alienated parents and children, it would be paramount to consider what confounding variables played a role in the study. Having children and alienated parents interact and engage with each other prior to the TPFF intervention means that the changes in attitude or supposed effectiveness of the program could be due to other causes, including this reconnecting before the start of the program.

Lastly, as discussed by Harman and colleagues in the article, the concern of harm is ever-present for scholars or other mental health professionals who do not endorse the concept of parental alienation (Harman et al., 2021). As Mercer mentions, the increased number of lawsuits of children adversely affected by parental alienation education/treatment programs cannot be dismissed (Mercer, 2021b). Harman's focus on the non-problematic behavior of the children during the program does not indicate that these children who experienced the program are not adversely affected or traumatized. Although no study has officially been conducted regarding the adverse effects of such programs, the presence of lawsuits toward these programs indicates some individuals have bad experiences and subsequent trauma. These lawsuits have highlighted issues of harm in these kinds of programs and these people's voices should not be ignored.

In H.L.J v. R.G.J., a 2017 custody case from Pennsylvania, the court-ordered psychologist of the mother and child referred them to engage in Gottlieb's Turning Points Program (*H.L.J v. R.G.J. Superior Court of Pennsylvania*, 2020). The case was such that the child was under the primary physical custody of the father and partial physical custody to the mother. They began to undergo reunification therapy before being referred to Gottlieb, and the child was experiencing anxiety to the point that she no longer wanted to meet with her mother. The individual conducting the reunification therapy, Dr. Adrian Quinn, opined that the child's rejection of the mother was influenced by the father. As a result, he recommended a higher level of care and referred them to Gottlieb. The father was opposed to the idea and argued that Gottlieb's methodology was not widely accepted and is opposed by a majority of her peers. Gottlieb was asked to testify in the case and the father argued that, as a result of the lack of evidence-based practice of her program, Gottlieb's entire testimony should be disregarded. However, because of the "liberal definition" of what qualifies one to be considered an expert in the Pennsylvania court, Gottlieb was still ultimately considered an expert in the case (*H.L.J v. R.G.J. Superior Court of Pennsylvania*, 2020). Gottlieb states that she believed it was important for the mother and the child to undergo intensive reunification therapy as well as that she found no signs of abuse within the relationship. However, it was not clear how Gottlieb was able to come to this conclusion. This led the father to remain in a difficult position: if the father did not support the mother's relationship with the child, the no contact period, as required by Gottlieb for TPFF, would be extended indefinitely. By extending the no-contact period indefinitely, one could question if this is also leading to alienating the other parent in the end.

Additional research that is present on Gottlieb's website are general articles written about Parental Alienation, in which details of her program and its scientific efficacy are not discussed (Reay, 2015; Warshak, 2010, 2015). From these articles that Gottlieb highlights on her website, we recognize that only two of the three are research studies (Reay, 2015; Warshak, 2010). Furthermore, there are two main concerns with each of these studies. First, both studies are from quite some time ago (2010 and 2012). Although this does not invalidate the proposed findings, this does not reflect the most recent research in the field and would require more recent follow-up. Second, both studies obtained a rather small sample size of 22–23 participants (Reay, 2015; Warshak, 2010). With such a minuscule sample size, it is difficult and scientifically misguided to generalize such results to the general public. These results can solely provide a preview of the effectiveness of the programs discussed in the articles.

Overall, we see the program can have its attraction with families struggling and facing difficult dynamics, bit it is not necessarily based on scientific research methods.

Given the information provided, the procedures of the program appear to be a form of informal therapy, with a total of approximately sixteen hours of formal therapy. It is also unclear what kind of therapeutic modality is being utilized in these three to four-hour daily sessions. The therapeutic modality used in sessions can likely vary from case to case; however, if this were the case, this should be discussed in the overview of the program.

Although Gottlieb has established the program to promote her methods of how to resolve parental alienation, there is only one published outcome study regarding the effectiveness of the program. Therefore, people are encouraged to engage in a program that, prior to 2021, did not have any scientific backing or validity. This is a great concern given the fundamental assumptions of parental alienation, such as the belief children must have contact with both parents for their psychological benefit, are weakly supported by evidence (Mercer, 2021a).

Thus, three main concerns arise surrounding this program. First, if an intense dispute occurs between parents, it is essential to explore how the parents came into this situation and how the child became involved in this dynamic. Second, it is important to determine what the concern of the child is. What exactly needs to change (e.g. difficult behavior, emotional approach)? This will help operationalize potential effectiveness of the program on a particular family. In essence, it is imperative to listen to the child. Whether such allegations were to be true or false, the reality is the child might still experience difficult reactions with a parent who has not been around them for a while. A relationship cannot be imposed on someone and, even if the child maintains misinformed beliefs of a parent, it is vital to consider the psychological impact of this process on the child. Exploring these adverse effects or potential risks could highlight the transparency of the program and provide further avenues of improvement for the future. Currently, the program is marketed as a family program; however, the focus tends to be on the satisfaction of the parents. It would be advised to have each parent of the child attend individual therapy before engaging in such a program. The child should also engage in individualized therapy for others to obtain further insight into the feelings and thoughts of the child through the litigation process. Third, the structure of TPFF relies on the absence of the "alienating parent" in the outings and aftermath of the program. Ultimately, it is vital to understand why Gottlieb concluded the "alienating" parent should not attend these outings and why this was the best method for reuniting the child and "rejected" parent. These explanations would provide a better understanding of the program as well as the reasoning behind the techniques and protocols.

Deutsch, Ward, Sullivan, and Friend's Overcoming Barriers

The Overcoming Barriers (OCB) Family Camp is an intensive treatment program designed for high-conflict families (Sullivan et al., 2010). According to Sullivan and colleagues as well as Judge and Deutsch (2010; 2016), the development of the camp came after an attempt to reunify a father and his children, which was sabotaged by the mother. This led Dr. Judge to work with the counselors to create a program that included all members of the family (Judge & Deutsch, 2016). An important element about OCB is that it specifies that it is only supposed to be used with families, "when the rejection [of a parent] has been determined to be unjustified by or disproportionate to the child's experience of the parent" (Judge & Deutsch, 2016, p. 133). However, according to the OCB website, Family Camp is currently canceled indefinitely due to a lack of appropriate funding for the resources needed to maintain it. Nevertheless, they are still offering training to mental health professionals, lawyers, and judges, as well as publishing books.

Referrals can be made by legal parties involved in the case, when both parents commit to children having a relationship with both parents. OCB is designed to be four to five days in length, however there is also an intensive two and a half to three-day immersion version (Judge & Deutsch, 2016). Each day contains interventions planned by psychologists (Sullivan et al., 2010). In the morning, groups are divided into children, the favored parents, and the "alienated" parents (Judge & Deutsch, 2016). This way there is support from people going through similar experiences; however, this has led to polarization of groups (Judge & Deutsch, 2016). OCB also included occasional groups of mixed parents, although there is no visible standardization of this (Judge & Deutsch, 2016). Counselors provide psychoeducation with themes of "goals and motivations; appropriate expectations and possibilities of change; identifying and correcting cognitive distortions; issues of fear, safety, overprotection, and under protection; strategies for coping with intense effect; and effective tools for direct communication" (Judge & Deutsch, 2016, p. 138). The groups are used as smaller, more controlled versions of life outside of camp. Group leaders also help parents translate activities to improve communication, emotional regulation, and their relationship with the child (Sullivan et al., 2010). This allows parents to practice being vulnerable and express emotions in a safer way (Sullivan et al., 2010). Groups for children focus on psycho-education, specifically through themes of "building group cohesion and trust; understanding different points of view; understanding how thoughts, feelings, and behaviors are related; identifying cognitive distortions; and changing behavior in small (or larger) increments" (Judge & Deutsch, 2016, p. 138). The goals for children's groups are to make the child's view of both parents less rigid such that they view each parent more realistically to ultimately fix their relationships with both parents (Sullivan et al., 2010).

The second portion of each day is when a mental health clinician works with each parent, parental figure, or the entire family unit. During these sessions, the clinicians focus aim to, "(1) address the dynamics that maintained their high level of interparental conflict; (2) structure, plan, and support the connections between the rejected parent and child; (3) address disputes in the parenting plan; and (4) discuss and recommend aftercare services" (Sullivan et al., 2010, p. 123). In these sessions, clinicians combine family systems therapy and concepts such as distortions, perspective-taking, desensitization, exposure therapy, suggestibility, and misperception (Judge & Deutsch, 2016). These techniques are quite diverse, and several of them require longer than five days to be utilized effectively. Judge and Deutsch discuss how it can be problematic if clients come in with preexisting therapists because they often take their client's "side" and do not look at the situation from a family systems lens, especially if they are treating their client for posttraumatic stress disorder (PTSD) symptoms due to marital abuse (2016). The first concern is the implication someone's individual therapist should be working for the entire family, even if that is not their client. This could lead to difficult dynamics in the therapeutic space. The second concern is if the client has PTSD from marital abuse, then rejection of the other parent by the child is justified and not eligible for OCB based on their requirements. Sullivan and colleagues report co-parenting sessions reflect high-conflict patterns they previously engaged in, and even with intensive individual counseling, many of these dyads did not find any resolution (2010).

The third portion of each day is the closing circle, where everyone in camp sits together, listens to announcements, and plans for the next day (Judge & Deutsch, 2016). The attendees practice new skills and observe each other in different situations (Judge & Deutsch, 2016). This helps perceptions of other family members' units by seeing more potential and humanizing them.

Milieu therapy is utilized to enhance the therapeutic experience (Sullivan et al., 2010). Milieu therapy is a treatment approach utilizing resources of a controlled environment (Raskin, 1976). Location and facilities are structured to encourage the separation of children from favored parents, connect the parents, allow children of similar age and gender to connect and support each other, as well as maximize staff support (Sullivan et al., 2010).

At the end of the program, there is a talent show called, "the Big Show" where everyone organizes into groups of their choice and performs. This is an opportunity for family members to see each other in different contexts and work successfully as a team (Judge & Deutsch, 2016). Then they hold the "final circle," where the whole camp gathers. During this time, everyone has a chance to write anonymous affirmations and put them in a box to be read out loud by staff. The staff also write an affirmation for each family. Before leaving, each family is set up with professionals outside the camp to continue the progress they have made. After everyone leaves, the staff all engage in a debriefing session (Judge & Deutsch, 2016). The program creators performed one study to test the efficacy and validity of the program. In *Overcoming parent-child contact problems: Family-based interventions for resistance, rejection, and alienation* by Judge and Deutsch, Michael Saini, Ph.D. coauthored a chapter that describes what should go into an evaluation of a program like OCB, however that was not the protocol that was followed (Judge & Deutsch, 2016). Contrastingly, a mixed-methods within-subjects design with no comparison group was used and included pre-intervention, post-intervention, and follow-up assessments (with no timeline mentioned) as well as qualitative interviews with the parents and the children (Judge & Deutsch, 2016). The only form of assessment used by family members was a self-report Likert-style questionnaire designed for parents, and only the parents filled it out all three times (Judge & Deutsch, 2016). The sample size for this study was 10 families, which consisted of 20 parents and 24 children, but only 13 of the children completed the survey even once (Judge & Deutsch, 2016). The other 11 participated in a qualitative interview; however, findings from that portion of the study are not available in the book (Judge & Deutsch, 2016). The authors acknowledge that they did not control for any outside factors that could impact the results of the study, which is a basic component of any reliable scientific research (Judge & Deutsch, 2016). To ensure that families receive the same treatment, the facilitators fill out a "fidelity checklist" (Judge & Deutsch, 2016). This checklist simply lists parts of the program and asks the responder to check 'yes' or 'no' regarding referral and screening factors, facilitator adherence, facilitator adherence, target population, location/setting, materials, delivery, dosage, and aftercare, but does not address treatment of participants or specific strategies utilized (Judge & Deutsch, 2016).

A follow-up study was later conducted entitled, *Strengthening Coparenting Relationships to Improve Strained Parent-Child Relationships: A Follow-Up Study of Parents' Experiences of Attending the OCB Program.* In this study, a link was sent anonymously to those who attended the camp (Saini, 2019). They had to meet inclusion criteria and provide informed consent. There was a sample size of 40 participants, with 57.1% mothers and 42.9% fathers (Saini, 2019). The sample was split exactly evenly between favored and rejected parents (Saini, 2019). However, 10.7% of the participants did not attend family camp but participated in services offered by OCB outside of that format (Saini, 2019). This study only used a qualitative survey as well as the Success of Interventions for Strained Relationships (SISR), which is a 15 question, Likert-style survey (Saini, 2019). Every participant only filled out the survey and SISR one time, with the time since they attended the camp ranging from six months to 10 years (Saini, 2019).

There were no statistically significant findings with the Overcoming Barriers Approach. The qualitative portion of this study demonstrated preconceived expectations parents and children had before attending camp greatly influenced their experience (Judge & Deutsch, 2016). The most valuable conclusion is the purpose of OCB is, "to plant seeds of hope and help families on the road to repairing strained relationships" and they acknowledge it is not feasible to completely fix these relationships in such a short time frame (Judge & Deutsch, 2016, p. 293).

In the follow-up study, Saini (2019) states that there was no difference in the results from the individual as well as the group format and this is why the results are combined; however, no statistics were provided to demonstrate this. Through qualitative analysis, Saini noted that 42.5% of participants did not find the program met their expectations and only 25% of participants found it did (Saini, 2019). Participants joined the program for a variety of reasons; therefore, whether or not it met their expectations is not a consistent measurement for the outcome of the program. Many people also reported that the courts either did not follow up nor utilize the information appropriately, which led to personal confusion and distress (Saini, 2019). Most parents indicated their understanding and ability to take responsibility for the problems within their relationship, as well as the impact on their children, improved since attending the camp (Saini, 2019). About half (48.1%) of parents reported the conflict in their relationship remained the same, and 25.9% reported there was more conflict than before (Saini, 2019). Quantitative results demonstrated 86.7% of participants reported improvements; however, this article only stated this refers to improvements in their view of each other, not the co-parenting relationship (Saini, 2019). Although developing an aftercare plan was part of the design of the program, only 67.9% reported this actually occurred (Saini, 2019). Within that 67.9%, many reported that there were problems maintaining it, whether that was the fault of the parents or the court (Saini, 2019).

Discussion

The structure and theory behind the OCB program have several strengths including that the program includes the entire family, and that they try to have a one-to-one ratio of staff to attendees (Saini, 2019). The training and qualifications of the staff that are around the participants are not specified in any detail, which is cause for concern. It does say that psychologists created the interventions; there is nothing written about who implements or supervises any of the interventions. This leaves a lot of room for inconsistency, as well as no way to ensure that the interventions are implemented correctly. If the people providing these interventions are not licensed psychologists, then there is also no way to ensure they would know how to handle complications when they undoubtedly arise. The description of the program is notably missing any way to avoid parental biases within the staff. There is a debrief at the end of the entire program; however, at that point, it could be considered too little too late. When working closely with people in such high conflict situations, it is difficult to avoid bias one way or the other; therefore, it is vital to address it before it causes any potential damage.

Even if the issues discussed above were addressed, the format of both studies does not yield reliable or informative results. In the 2016 study, the sample size is very small and children did not have the opportunity to discuss their experiences more than once. This makes it impossible to discuss long-term effects of the program on these children. Furthermore, as some families are court involved, participants saying what was needed for their desired outcomes is additional risk to the research. Another threat to the validity is 10.7% of participants did not attend the camp and participated in a different intensive program (Saini, 2019). If these participants did not attend, then their results cannot speak to the efficacy of the camp. The sample is not generalizable, as Saini reports 53.8% had a university degree and 80% of them earned more than $100,000 a year (2019). These figures do not reflect most of the population. Although the second study obtained a larger sample size, external variables were not addressed or eliminated. Results were also not clearly operationalized. The information from qualitative surveys used in both studies did not have evident goals for the conclusions. They helped clarify the parent's individual feelings about the program, however, they did not demonstrate the efficacy of it or how it helped the children (Judge & Deutsch, 2016; Saini, 2019).

No children were included in the 2019 study which can be seen as incredibly troubling, considering the point of the camp is about the relationship with their parents and the good of the child. The point of the camp should be to help the parents to be able to effectively parent their children without causing any more harm to the children (Judge & Deutsch, 2016). The children's view of their parents and the treatment they are receiving should be the focal point of determining the effectiveness of this program. Since the OCB program does recognize that it cannot cause this change on its own, it should have more emphasis on maintaining the aftercare programs as well. Although there are complications during court proceedings, implementing, and participating in these aftercare programs should be mandatory. This should be the case as it was part of the design of the program. Although the theory behind the OCB camp is solid, there need to be structural changes and efficacy testing if the camp were to be continued in the future.

Conclusion

Although each program discussed has its limitations, programs which focus on parental alienation are limited in terms of research foundation. The lack of research in the field of parental alienation makes it challenging to establish programs supported by scientific evidence. The focal point of future studies should be on the children and the impact these programs have on them, as opposed to the parents involved in litigation. As the concept of parental alienation is questioned in psychology, programs catered to this notion should be approached with great caution. The consequences of engaging in these programs could be financially and emotionally detrimental to families, especially amid abuse allegations. Furthermore, the child would likely experience more emotional difficulty whist in contact with the potential abuser than not being in contact with them. If these programs intend to operate in the future, it would be advised the respective directors conduct further scientific research to substantiate their claims, procedures, and program efficacy. By conducting further research into these programs, individuals involved in litigations can have a holistic and better understanding of the potential advantages as well as disadvantages of engaging in reunification or educational programs.

Disclosure of interest

Although there are no conflicts to report, it is important to note that Elena Andreopoulos and Alison Wexler completed their internships at the Institute of Violence, Abuse, and Trauma (IVAT) under the guidance of Dr. Robert A. Geffner (July 2020-August 2021).

Acknowledgments

The authors would like to greatly thank Dr. Robert Geffner for the initial guidance on this article and the space created to discuss these ideas. Thank you also to Dr. Jean Mercer for the additional insight and support for this work. Lastly, thank you to all the editors, including Dr. Brittany Crowell, for the guidance on the publication process.

References

Baker, A., & Fine, P. (2007). *Adult children of parental alienation syndrome: Breaking the ties that bind*. New York: Norton

Bernet, W. (2010). Definitions and goals. In *Parental alienation, DSM-5, and ICD-11* (pp. 3–8). Charles C Thomas.

Brainerd, C. J., & Poole, D. A. (1997). Long-term survival of children's false memories: A review. *Learning and Individual Differences, 9*(2), 125–151. https://doi.org/10.1016/S1041-6080(97)90003-0

Chan, J. C. K., O'Donnell, R., & Manley, K. D. (2022). Warning weakens retrieval-enhanced suggestibility only when it is given shortly after misinformation: The critical importance of timing. *Journal of Experimental Psychology: Applied, 139*, 83. https://doi.org/10.1037/xap0000394

Darnall, D. (2011). The psychosocial treatment of parental alienation. *Child and Adolescent Psychiatric Clinics of North America, 20*(3), 479–494. https://doi.org/10.1016/j.chc.2011.03.006

Faller, K. C. (1984). Is the child victim of sexual abuse telling the truth? *Child Abuse & Neglect, 8*(4), 473–481. https://doi.org/10.1016/0145-2134(84)90029-2

Faller, K. C. (2007). Coaching children about sexual abuse: A pilot study of professionals' perceptions. *Child Abuse & Neglect, 31*(9), 947–959. https://doi.org/10.1016/j.chiabu.2007.05.004

Gardner, R. A. (1992). *The parental alienation syndrome: A guide for mental health and legal professionals*. Creative Therapeutics.

Gottlieb, L. J. (2012). *The parental alienation syndrome: A family therapy and collaborative systems approach to amelioration*. Charles C Thomas.

Gottlieb, L. J. (2013). The application of structural family therapy to the treatment of parental alienation. In A. J. Baker & S. R. Sauber (Eds.), *Working with alienated children and families: A clinical guidebook* (pp. 209–231).

Gottlieb, L. J. (2020a). *Children are harmed when professionals reject science* (Vol. *20*). End Parental Alienation. https://endparentalalienation.weebly.com

Gottlieb, L. J. (2020b). *Reasons for the apology letter from the alienating parent* (p. 6). Family Access Fighting for Children's Rights. https://www.familyaccessfightingforchildrensrights.com/uploads/2/6/5/0/26505602/reasons_for_the_apology_letter.pdf

Gottlieb, L. J. (2021a). *Reunification therapy for severe parental alienation or for an unreasonably disrupted parent-child relationship* (pp. 1–17). Turning Points for Families. https://turningpoints4families.weebly.com/uploads/2/2/5/4/22545256/07-12-2020_tpff_treatment_protocol_x_4_6_18_ent_protocol_for_severe_alieantion_rejection.pdf

Gottlieb, L. J. (2021b). Turning *points* for *families*. https://turningpoints4families.weebly.com/

H.L.J v. R.G.J. Superior Court of Pennsylvania. (2020). https://www.casemine.com/judgement/us/5f291aa64653d02f6f5f90c1

Harman, J. J., Saunders, L., & Afifi, T. (2021). Evaluation of the Turning Points for Families (TPFF) program for severely alienated children. *Journal of Family Therapy*, 1–20. https://doi.org/10.1111/1467-6427.12366

Joshi, A. (Ed.). (2021). *Litigating parental alienation: evaluating and presenting an effective case in Court*. ABA, American Bar Association, Family Law Section.

Judge, A., & Deutsch, R. M. (Eds.). (2016). *Overcoming parent-child contact problems: Family-based interventions for resistance, rejection, and alienation*. Oxford University Press.

Long Island Backstory. (2018). *Linda Gottlieb, LMFT, LCSW-R a World Renowned Expert In Parental Alienation On Long Island Backstory [Video]*. Long Island Backstory. https://www.youtube.com/watch?v=QasBM1ei4NI&ab_channel=LongIslandBackstory

Lorandos, D., Bernet, W., & Sauber, S. R. (2013). Foundations of parental alienation: historical, scientific, and legal. In *Parental alienation: The handbook for mental health and legal professionals* (pp. 289–535). Charles C. Thomas.

Lyon, T. D., & Dorado, J. S. (2008). Truth induction in young maltreated children: The effects of oath-taking and reassurance on true and false disclosures. *Child Abuse & Neglect*, *32*(7), 738–748. https://doi.org/10.1016/j.chiabu.2007.08.008

Mercer, J. (2021a). Critiquing assumptions about parental alienation: Part 2. Causes of psychological harms. *Journal of Family Trauma, Child Custody & Child Development*, 1–18. https://doi.org/10.1080/26904586.2021.1957058

Mercer, J. (2021b). Not on the levels: Harman says she evaluated Turning Points. Child Myths Blogspot. https://childmyths.blogspot.com/2021/09/not-on-levels-harman-says-she-evaluated.html

O'Donohue, W., Cummings, C., & Willis, B. (2018). The frequency of false allegations of child sexual abuse: A critical review. *Journal of Child Sexual Abuse*, *27*(5), 459–475. https://doi.org/10.1080/10538712.2018.1477224

Raskin, D. E. (1976). Milieu therapy reexamined. *Comprehensive Psychiatry*, *17*(6), 695–701. https://doi.org/10.1016/0010-440X(76)90017-1

Reay, K. M. (2015). Family reflections: A promising therapeutic program designed to treat severely alienated children and their family system. *The American Journal of Family Therapy*, *43*(2), 197–207. https://doi.org/10.1080/01926187.2015.1007769

Ruck, M. D. (1996). Why children think they should tell the truth in court: Developmental considerations for the assessment of competency. *Legal and Criminological Psychology*, *1*(1), 103–116. https://doi.org/10.1111/j.2044-8333.1996.tb00310.x

Rush, E. (2014). Children's true and false disclosures of transgressions: Balancing costs and benefits of a novel interviewing technique. In *Dissertation Abstracts International: Section B: The Sciences and Engineering*. University of California.

Saini, M. (2019). Strengthening coparenting relationships to improve strained parent–child relationships: A follow-up study of parents' experiences of attending the overcoming barriers program. *Family Court Review*, *57*(2), 217–230. https://doi.org/10.1111/fcre.12405

Starns, J. J., & Hicks, J. L. (2005). Source dimensions are retrieved independently in multidimensional monitoring asks. *Journal of Experimental Psychology: Learning, Memory, and Cognition*, *31*(6), 1213–1220.

Sullivan, M. J., Ward, P. A., & Deutsch, R. M. (2010). Overcoming barriers family camp: A program for high-conflict divorced families where a child is resisting contact with a parent. *Family Court Review*, *48*(1), 116–135. https://doi.org/10.1111/j.1744-1617.2009.01293.x

Warshak, R. A. (2010). Family bridges: Using insights from social science to reconnect parents and alienated children. *Family Court Review*, *48*(1), 48–80. https://doi.org/10.1111/j.1744-1617.2009.01289.x

Warshak, R. A. (2015). Ten parental alienation fallacies that compromise decisions in court and in therapy. *Professional Psychology: Research and Practice*, *46*(4), 235–249. https://doi.org/10.1037/pro0000031

Index

Note: Figures are indicated by *italics*. Tables are indicated by **bold**